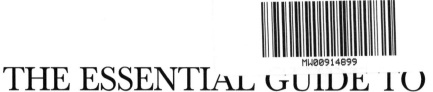
THE ESSENTIAL GUIDE TO

OZONE

THERAPY

FOR ANIMALS

HOW OXYGEN DEFICIENCY IS KILLING OUR ANIMALS AND WHAT TO DO ABOUT IT

Jonathan Lowe

Independently Published

This book contains advice and information relating to veterinary health care. It should be used to supplement rather than replace the advice of your veterinarian or another trained veterinary health professional. If you know or suspect that your pet has a health problem, it is recommended that you seek your veterinarian's advice before embarking on any medical program or treatment. All efforts have been made to assure the accuracy of the information contained in this book as of the date of publication. The author disclaims liability for any medical outcomes that may occur as a result of applying the methods suggested in this book.

FIRST EDITION

ISBN 979-8-37-508896-9

For information, please write to info@o3vets.com

To Kimberly,
the love of my life for over twenty years

Contents

Introduction

I am a big fan of modern medicine. I appreciate living in a country that gives me access to that medicine. As an advocate for a treatment that has been labeled "alternative," it's natural to adopt an us-against-the-world mentality and view conventional medicine as the enemy.

It's not.

Through the years, I have known numerous people who rail against current best practices in medicine to deal with infections, autoimmune conditions, cancer, and more. They will often use more natural, less-invasive treatments to deal with minor conditions for themselves and their pets, but, when they are diagnosed with cancer or living with chronic infection, they cave and undergo the same treatments they initially mocked.

Of course, there are many who stay the course and stick with an anti-cancer diet, herbs, and nonconventional treatments. So which approach is best? How do we navigate health problems? What will you do when disease affects you, your patients, or your pets?

In 2007, I moved my family to Bolivia. We were exposed to parasites and diseases we had never experienced before. We had two little girls under the age of three, and both of them ended up with parasites. At that time in our lives, my wife, Kimberly, and I had not yet been introduced to integrative treatments (like ozone therapy). We followed the advice of our doctors without question. Some of that advice was superb, but there was a fundamental flaw in it. Their advice flowed out of a worldview that accepted pharmaceuticals as the primary answer to our problems. This meant that every year, regardless of whether it was necessary or not, we and many of our friends would put our children on a round of antibiotics to rid them of known or potential parasites.

Here's the fundamental problem: We all want to live a lifestyle that allows us to eat what we want, exercise if we feel like it, and still maintain optimal health. When a health concern arises, we want an easy fix. We want it to be fast, cheap, and easy. That's the bottom line. I want it. You want it. We all want it. We like the antibiotic route because it's easy and allows us to keep living in relative comfort without too many interruptions. If you are one of those who has pushed against that ideology, then you are part of a very small minority.

Pharmaceutical companies sell it, educational institutions teach it, doctors prescribe it, insurance companies pay for it, and the general public buys it. That's the cycle, and we're all part of it.

But what happens when the cycle is disrupted? What happens when someone starts to question whether the basic presuppositions upon which our healthcare system rests are actually true? What happens when someone is brave enough to swim upstream and do the hard work to maintain health by supporting their God-given immune system—to eat in ways that provide vital nutrients to our cells and exercise to strengthen their cardiovascular systems and increase oxygenation?

I'll admit, although I am a fan of modern medicine, I also believe that we need to make some drastic changes for ourselves and our pets.

We need to adopt healthy lifestyles.

We need to practice medicine that addresses animals holistically.

We need to introduce difficult changes.

We need to take responsibility for our own actions.

We need to accept that there are things we don't know.

We need to be proactive instead of reactive when it comes to the health of our animals.

I could go on.

Sometimes a treatment comes along that heralds a system's biological approach to medicine. A treatment like this can be incredibly valuable. This book is about such a treatment called ozone therapy.

With the extraordinary rise of chronic diseases and the unprecedented use of pharmaceuticals that tend to suppress symptoms rather than get to root causes, I believe that ozone therapy will play a critical role in restoring the health of our animals. I am not alone in that sentiment.

I met Dr. Margo Roman in 2013. She is an incredibly dedicated and courageous veterinarian who lives in the Boston area. Dr. Roman practices integrative medicine, is politically active, and stands up for what she believes in. She got her start in the 1970s and immediately began to look for answers in unconventional places. I credit Dr. Roman with much of the success of my company, O3Vets, because it was Dr. Roman who gave me real insight into how ozone could be used in veterinary practice. She encouraged me to develop equipment and education that would help the veterinarian.

During an interview with her, Dr. Roman stated that she did not know how to practice medicine without ozone therapy. At first, I didn't believe her statement, but after visiting her practice, it's true. She really wouldn't know how to practice medicine without ozone therapy.

Dr. Marlene Siegel is a thought leader among veterinarians and a good friend of mine. When I first met her, she told me she wanted the whole ozone therapy setup. Cost wasn't even in the equation for Dr. Siegel because she believed that ozone therapy would make an incredible difference in the animals she treated. Over the years, her hunch proved true. Dr. Siegel said the following at a past ozone training class, "Ozone is one of the best tools that I've ever integrated into my practice and has helped me provide patients with the best outcome possible."

There have been a few books written about ozone therapy, but, to my knowledge, this will be the first practical book written about ozone therapy for animals. By reading this book, you will discover three basic areas:

1) What ozone therapy is
2) How it benefits animals
3) How to get started

As I said above, I intend to be intensely practical. By the end of this book, I don't want you to just say, "Hey, I know what ozone therapy is now." Instead, I want you to say, "Hey, I know how ozone therapy applies to animals, and I can actually do this!" At the same time, there will likely be some information that will be difficult for the average pet owner to sift through. I desire to both provide the veterinarian with a valuable resource for understanding and implementing ozone therapy and make the information accessible and useful for a pet owner as well.

Chapter 1

How Oxygen Deficiency and Inflammation Are Killing Our Animals

All chronic pain, suffering and diseases are caused by a lack of oxygen at the cell level.

DR. ARTHUR C. GUYTON

There's a one-in-four chance that your dog will get cancer and a one-in-five chance that your cat will get cancer. Over half of our dogs and cats are overweight or obese. For cats over ten years old, 30% experience chronic kidney disease. Autoimmune diseases are on the rise. Maintaining optimal health in our pets becomes increasingly difficult in a fast-paced world governed by the need for an immediate solution to deeply rooted issues.

"Give me a list of items that are essential for good health," I said to a group of veterinary students at Michigan State University.

"Nutrition."

"Water."

"Sleep."

"Exercise."

The list may vary slightly, but whenever I ask this question, the answers are basically the same because we all need the same things to survive and thrive. "What about oxygen?" I asked. "In fact, I think that within the next five minutes, I can prove that oxygen is the single-most-important nutrient for us and our animals. We're all going to hold our breath for five minutes. Are you ready? Go!" Of course, the experiment only lasted a few seconds because we all recognize it's an exercise in futility, but it proves an important point. Oxygen is assumed. It's taken for granted, and not only by veterinary students but by almost everyone, including many doctors. If you were to lose oxygen for even a few minutes, you would die. Our bodies and our animals' bodies have been designed to utilize oxygen every second of every day. Behind the scenes, an unknown number of biological processes including redox signaling, the creation of ATP, and protein synthesis are taking place to keep us alive and healthy.

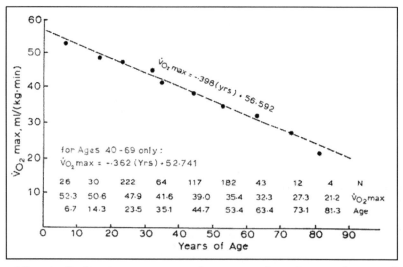

Figure 1: Longitudinal variations in maximal oxygen intake with age and activity. J. App. Physiol. 33(6): 805-807. 1972.

As our bodies age, our ability to utilize oxygen decreases. The same phenomenon holds true for chronic disease. There is a general rule that the unhealthier we are, the less effective our body is at utilizing oxygen. As oxygen utilization decreases, normal biological functions suffer, creating a cascade effect into a vicious cycle of dysregulation. In fact, decreased oxygen utilization is what leads to chronic inflammation, mitochondrial breakdown, and eventually death if not corrected. This is exactly why Dr. Guyton said, "All chronic pain, suffering and diseases are caused by a lack of oxygen at the cell level." And Dr. Guyton was no slouch. He wrote the textbook for medical physiology that many still use. If Dr. Guyton thought that oxygen was *the* most critical building block of health, why is it not our primary goal to ensure that we take care of oxygen utilization?

When I use the term "oxygen utilization," I am referring to the efficiency of a cell to convert the energy contained in an oxygen molecule into usable energy to carry out physiological processes.

Dr. Stephen Levine is a renowned molecular biologist and the author of *Oxygen Deficiency*. In that book he makes this incredible statement, "In all serious disease conditions we find low oxygen level. Oxygen deficiency in our bodies' tissues is an indicator for disease. Hypoxia, or lack of oxygen in the tissues, is the fundamental cause for all degenerative disease."

Dr. Guyton and Dr. Levine are right. Finding the key and unlocking the door to oxygen utilization is crucial, but it's not that easy.

In his book *Principles and Applications of Ozone Therapy*, Dr. Frank Shallenberger points out that "there are many factors that act to decrease oxygen utilization. These include: decreased lipolysis, decreased fatty acid metabolism, nutritional deficiencies, sleep deprivation, hormonal deficiencies, toxicity, infections, hypoxia, decreased methylation, ischemia, stress, inflammation, and hypoglycemia." Anyone who has cared for animals for any length of time knows that maintaining health is never as simple as one change or one treatment. There is no silver bullet, but there are critical components that must be in place.

One central area for optimal oxygen uptake and utilization is exercise. Without exercise, our health and the health of our animals quickly deteriorate. Our muscles, including those needed for breathing, will shrink and weaken. Small amounts of activity will become difficult, and we will feel short of breath. Eventually, even the smallest tasks will seem impossible. For most, we can fight this downward spiral just by staying active, but what about those who are aging or sick?

In a review published in the clinical section of the *Journal of Gerontology*, Martin Burtscher proposes the following:

> Cardiorespiratory fitness (aerobic exercise capacity) is one of the most important prerequisites for successful aging in human beings and depends on adequate oxygen transport by the respiratory and circulatory systems from environmental air to the working muscles and the efficient utilization of oxygen by the mitochondria. A linear dose-response relation between aerobic exercise capacity, morbidity, mortality, and quality of life is well documented. The process of normal aging is associated with a variable reduction in functional capacity of the main organs involved in oxygen delivery and utilization. Specific exercise training programs, considering the state of cardiorespiratory health and physical activity, are the most important and almost the only effective intervention to avoid or to

break the circulus vitiosus (vicious cycle), thereby promoting quality and expectancy of life in aging humans.[1]

In other words, our health is fully dependent on our body's ability to take in, break down, and utilize oxygen. And one of the only ways to maintain health so that our body does this is through exercise.

I'll admit, the only exercise that I like to do involves chasing a ball—basketball, baseball, football, volleyball, spike ball, soccer, bocci ball (okay, bocci ball probably doesn't fall into the category of exercise), but chasing a ball is the only way that I've been able to enjoy exercise.

And what about our animals? An animal in the wild gets plenty of exercise. They are forced into it if they want to survive. But think of a Great Dane living in an apartment in New York City or a Golden Retriever who doesn't get a daily walk, much less three walks per day. Could it be that lack of exercise is a significant factor in the deteriorating health and onset of chronic diseases in our pets?

Dr. Judith Shoemaker is a respected veterinarian with over 40 years of clinical experience. When I spoke with her a few years back, she made this statement, "I talk about ozone as being like 40 minutes of exercise in a syringe." While there's a lot more to ozone therapy that we'll unpack later in this book, this concept will help in understanding what ozone therapy is.

At this point, you may be thinking, "So is ozone therapy just for inactive animals?" The answer is no. Ozone therapy is of great importance for animals along the entire spectrum of health. The important takeaway is that ozone therapy can have a significant impact on health through modifying how the body utilizes oxygen.

I met Dr. Gerald Buchoff at a veterinary conference in 2016. I found out that he used ozone therapy, and so I decided to interview him. When I asked him what he would say to a veterinarian who might reject the idea of using ozone as a therapeutic tool, he responded, "I believe that if you're not using ozone, you need to. There are a lot of modalities out there, and we can't have all of them, but I feel like ozone is one of the most basic. What do animals need? They need hydration—no veterinarian would not have IV fluids—and oxygen. It's one of the basic needs for an animal. It just seems logical that you would need to deliver that to the patient, and there's no easier way to do that than by using ozone therapy."

A well-known treatment called Hyperbaric Oxygen Therapy (HBOT) was popularized in the 1930s to treat Navy divers suffering from decompression sickness. As this treatment evolved, it was used to treat wounds, concussions, tumors, and damaged muscles by bringing oxygen-rich plasma to oxygen-starved tissue. This process can, among other things, dramatically decrease inflammation and improve vascular flow. Many high-profile athletes like LeBron James, Cristiano Ronaldo, and Michael Phelps have used this technology to help their bodies recover from the stress of rigorous activity.

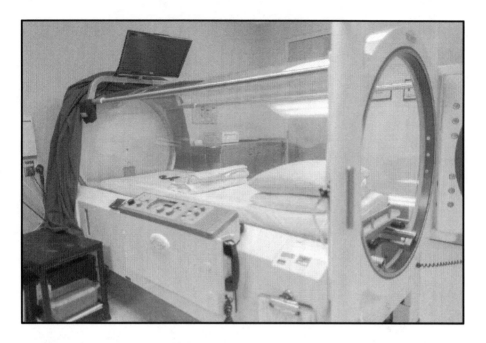

I spoke to a vet once who likened ozone therapy to "an internal hyperbaric chamber." I like this comparison because it gives people who are familiar with HBOT a category within which to understand ozone therapy. But the comparison falls short of what ozone really does. While HBOT is helpful in a number of circumstances and can deliver oxygen to an area, it cannot address underlying root causes of oxygen deficiency. And that is what ozone therapy is all about.

BLOOD OXYGEN TESTING

Today, veterinarians use a simple pulse oximetry meter to test blood oxygen levels. It may be tempting to think that we could simply use this technology or even blood samples to ascertain the levels of oxygen in our blood and determine whether we need to perform ozone therapy. While knowing blood oxygen levels can be helpful in some cases, it fails to show the complete picture. Most importantly, these tests cannot show how efficient our body is in *utilizing* the oxygen in the blood. The ultimate indication of efficient oxygen utilization is how much gets into the mitochondria, which is a much tougher measurement to get.

INFLAMMATION

Inflammation is a good thing. Well, let me rephrase that. Inflammation is a necessary evil. It is the body's response to injury and a vital part of the healing cascade. If pathogens, injuries, and sickness didn't exist, then inflammation wouldn't either, but until God finally makes all things right, inflammation must play a role if we and our animals want to survive.

We identify inflammation by five primary signs: redness, swelling, heat, pain, and loss of function. The two major categories of inflammation are acute and chronic. Acute inflammation usually lasts only a few hours to a few days and is often caused by trauma. As a result of the trauma, the body sends fluid, including a variety of white blood cells, from blood vessels to the surrounding tissue, destroying pathogens and healing the injury.

In contrast, chronic inflammation is rarely a good thing. It may start with the same cellular actions as acute inflammation, but it lingers for months or years. The body sounds the alarm and calls for troops to come to defend the body. But even when the threat is neutralized, the immune system continues to fight and begins to attack the body that it originally intended to defend.

Inflammation has been likened to fire. In the right location and intensity, fire keeps us warm and safe, but even a small out-of-control fire can do significant damage. Similarly, the low-grade inflammation that exists in chronically ill people and animals can destroy healthy cells and cause a cascade of health concerns. Some of the diseases linked to excessive inflammation are asthma, cancer, COPD, chronic pain, Type 2 diabetes, IBS, heart disease, and autoimmune conditions like arthritis, lupus, and scleroderma.

If I don't say something here about how important it is to prevent unnecessary inflammation through lifestyle choices, then my friend Dr. Siegel would be sorely disappointed. The reality is that consistent exercise, healthy eating, good sleep, and managing weight and stress in our pets will go a long way toward keeping them healthy.

I have had the privilege of meeting many wonderful veterinarians who have written extensively on these issues. Among them are Dr. Gary Richter who wrote *The Ultimate Pet Health Guide*, Dr. Barbara Royal who wrote *The Royal Treatment*, and Dr. Karen Becker who wrote *The Forever Dog*. Pick up any of these books and you'll discover some crucial information that can be useful to both veterinarians and pet owners alike. Regardless of how careful you or your clients are with promoting a healthy lifestyle, animals are still at risk of developing a chronic disease.

Poor oxygen utilization and chronic inflammation are two massive areas that affect health on a cellular level and lead to a cascade of chronic diseases. In chapter three we're going to deal with how ozone therapy works to increase oxygen utilization and reduce inflammation.

SUMMARY

As we consider the implications of this chapter, there are a few key truths to keep in mind:

- The most important key to successful aging in our pets is exercise.
- Lack of oxygen at the cellular level is the root of all known disease.
- Optimizing oxygen utilization is foundational to an animal's health.
- Adequate oxygen blood levels are not synonymous with adequate oxygen utilization.
- Chronic inflammation is a problem linked to many diseases.

These points should move us to action. If you work in a veterinary office, you must have treatments that address the root causes of poor oxygen utilization. Protocols that you have developed for specific disease processes should be adapted. Training for employees should take place to teach these concepts, and, ultimately, the client needs to know why taking care of the underlying inflammation and oxygen deficiency is so important.

If you care for an animal, you need to make sure they are getting enough exercise. You also need to find a veterinarian (even if it's through telemedicine) who understands these concepts and is able to address these issues.

Chapter 2

Ozone as a Therapy... Really?

"Ozone is a toxic gas with no known useful medical application in specific, adjunctive, or preventive therapy. In order for ozone to be effective as a germicide, it must be present in a concentration far greater than that which can be safely tolerated by man and animals."[2]

We might as well start with the elephant in the room. The FDA doesn't like ozone therapy. The really disturbing part of the statement made by the FDA in 1976 is that they haven't been willing to change it even though an incredible amount of scientific evidence shows that they are dead wrong. If you take a close look at the statement above, the FDA claims that, "In order for ozone to be effective as a germicide, it must be present in a concentration far greater than that which can be safely tolerated by man and animals." In my humble opinion, there are no words in the English language strong enough to communicate just how misleading and ignorant that statement is. As we'll see in the next chapter, the germicidal activity of ozone is not the mechanism by which it's working when infused into the body and, to my knowledge, it never was the proposed mechanism unless we are dealing with the external application.

Just like my stance on modern medicine, I respect the FDA and what they were *intended* to do. I also believe that somewhere along the way they lost their true north and succumbed to the manipulation of pharmaceutical and insurance companies. What was initially designed to protect the American people from harmful and ineffective treatments and medications has turned into a lobbyist's Candy Land—a game of epic proportions that includes shortcuts and secret passages for the rich and powerful but a slow and meandering journey for the approval of treatments like ozone therapy.

The FDA's position is not only one of ignorance but of superiority as well. While many of the studies conducted on ozone therapy are not tightly controlled and may be open to bias, there are stacks that are tightly controlled. In this country, we tend to look at studies that come from other countries with suspicion, as if the United States is the only place where science is taken seriously. Unfortunately, there are other, less developed countries who take their cues from the USA thinking that if Americans reject something, it must be bad, and if we accept something, then it must be good. We have a responsibility to our own country and to the world to set an example.

I want to be careful not to throw the baby out with the bath water because I know that we do a lot of good, but the problem of human greed is always in the picture, and our medical system is no different—from hospitals to insurance companies to individual practice owners and everyone in between. When a drug company is able to throw millions of dollars into ensuring that their product is positioned correctly, they have the upper hand. When lobbyists are paid big bucks to build relationships with key people and drive the agenda of the pharma company forward, it comes as no surprise that they get what they want. We like to imagine that research is unbiased, the doctor is superhuman, and the pharmaceutical company really does want to find a cure. The fact is that most research is funded in one way or another by pharmaceutical companies that highlight the information they want available and cover up the bad and call it a "trade secret." We all need to stand accountable and be part of the solution instead of part of the problem. The bottom line is that the FDA got it wrong, but until there is sufficient pressure on them from lobbyists, there is no real reason for them to revise their position on ozone therapy. The last time I checked, there aren't any ozone therapy companies that have the finances for lobbyists or the desire to take on the FDA.

But I will grant the FDA this: ozone is lethal. I'm not kidding. If you were to turn on your ozone generator and pump it into your lungs at high concentrations, it wouldn't take long before you would be toast. Don't do that.

I have often asked the question, "What comes to mind when you hear the word 'ozone?'" Two things are often mentioned, and they're never medical in nature. The first is smog or pollution. Ozone is considered a pollutant because it can have a negative effect on our lungs. The definition of pollution is, "The presence in or introduction into the environment of a substance or thing that has harmful or poisonous effects." That is the bad side of ozone. If you breathe in high enough concentrations for long enough, it is harmful. The Environmental Protection Agency (EPA) stated the following about smog:

> When inhaled, ozone can damage the lungs. Relatively low amounts can cause chest pain, coughing, shortness of breath, and throat irritation. Ozone may also worsen

chronic respiratory diseases such as asthma and compromise the ability of the body to fight respiratory infections. People vary widely in their susceptibility to ozone.[3]

Those affected by asthma, COPD, or similar diseases are particularly susceptible to the negative effects of inhaled ozone. In an article entitled "Effects of Air Pollutants on Airway Diseases," Lee et al. 2021, says:

> Ozone is highly reactive and oxidizes proteins and lipids in the fluid-lined compartment of the lung. This initiates inflammation and increases lung permeability, via cytotoxic mediators including pro-inflammatory cytokines, ROS, and nitrogen intermediates such as peroxynitrite. The primary targets for ozone are the distal structures of the lung, including the terminal bronchioles, bronchiole–alveolar duct junction, and proximal alveolar regions. Acute inhalation of ozone causes structural alterations in the lung, including disruption of the alveolar epithelial barrier, which lead to alveolar epithelial type II cell hypertrophy and hyperplasia. The recruitment of inflammatory cells into the lung following ozone exposure can also damage tissue via the release of toxic mediators (e.g., cytokines, ROS, nitrogen species, and proteolytic enzymes) from activated macrophages and neutrophils.[4]

Basically, the lack of sufficient antioxidants in the lung lining causes excessive inflammation. Let's just put this to rest before it becomes an issue. The inhalation of ozone gas is NOT one of the ways that we can safely administer ozone, but there are many safe, easy, and effective ways to administer it. We'll talk about those methods more in chapter five.

The ozone layer is the second area that people identify when asked what comes to mind when they hear the word "ozone." We think of the ozone layer depleting, and we know it's a bad thing, but most people don't know much about it. Because ozone has a largely negative connotation in the back of our minds somewhere, sadly, that connotation affects how people perceive ozone therapy. I want to encourage you to put down what you know about smog and the ozone layer and judge ozone therapy through an unbiased lens. Allow it to stand or fall according to the following criteria:

- Has it been proven safe as a medical treatment?
- Has it been proven effective as a medical treatment?

Safety and efficacy are the criteria that allow us to use a modality with confidence or not. Instead of looking solely to friends, trusted colleagues, or anecdotal information, we're going to discover what the scientific studies show and base our opinion on reality.

WHAT IS OZONE

Instead of providing a long-winded definition, here's a simple, easy description of ozone:

- A pale-blue gas made up of three oxygen atoms sharing electrons
- A powerful oxidizer and a reactive form of oxygen
- A distinctly pungent-smelling substance that resembles chlorine

Ozone is good. Without it, we would die. It's sunscreen for the Earth. Unfortunately, we hear a lot about the evils of ozone and how harmful it is to our health. We never hear about how it acts as a chemical cleanser for pollutants in the atmosphere. While we do need to discuss the dangers of ozone, I also want you to be aware that without it, we would be in big trouble.[5]

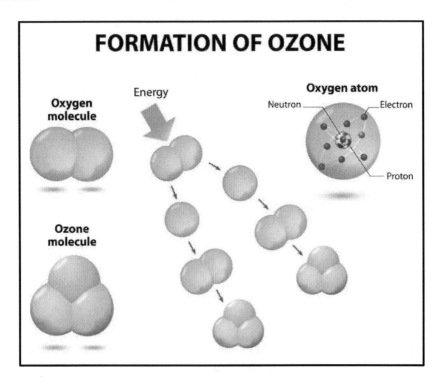

FORMATION OF OZONE

Oxygen molecule

Energy

Oxygen atom

Neutron

Electron

Proton

Ozone molecule

Ozone exists in small quantities near the Earth's surface where it can be harmful to plants, animals, and humans above 0.1 parts per million (ppm) and in the stratosphere in larger quantities where it protects us from harmful ultraviolet radiation. The oxygen atoms that combine to make up ozone don't share electrons well, which makes ozone unstable. Because of this, ozone quickly breaks down and reverts back to oxygen. Practically, this means that we can't store it for very long. When referring to ozone storage, the term "half-life" is used. Half-life is the amount of time it takes for ozone to lose half its potency. The half-life of ozone in air is about two hours. For example, if we have 50 μg/ml of ozone when we create it, after two hours we'll have 25 μg/ml if we keep that ozone in the same confined space. In a sterile fluid, the half-life of ozone is about 30-

40 minutes. That's why it's important to generate the ozone right before it is used. There are some exceptions to this that will be discussed in a later chapter.

Whether used in industrial or medical applications, ozone needs to be measured. In an industrial setting, this is usually done by using parts per million (ppm). This measurement is based on mass to mass or volume to volume whereas measurements in μg/ml are based on mass to volume ratios.

Here's the novice's guide to understanding this measurement: in ozone gas, 1 μg/ml is equivalent to 467 ppm[6], however, when dissolved into a fluid, it would be different.

Since we won't be using ppm in our medical settings, we're not going to talk about this measurement. It would get boring.

In the veterinary clinic, we use micrograms per milliliter (μg/ml) or milligrams per liter (mg/l) as the most common way to measure the concentration of ozone. These two measurements are equal, so don't let that trip you up—1 μg/ml is equal to 1 mg/l. This is a weight-based measurement that tells us how much ozone there is in a defined area compared to the total volume of that area. For example, if we draw up a 60 ml syringe of ozone at 50 μg/ml, we know that for each milliliter (ml) of space in the syringe, there will be 50 micrograms of ozone. Is it important to remember this? Probably not. But it is a good idea to at least try understanding some of these things so we can speak intelligently when clients or others ask questions. One practical note here is that, when ozone is created, most of what is drawn up into a syringe is actually oxygen. You will see some scientific literature using the term "oxygen/ozone" when referring to ozone therapy because only a small percentage (typically 2-5%) of the entire volume of gas in a syringe is actually ozone, and the rest is oxygen.

This is how it is supposed to be, and this doesn't diminish the efficacy of the treatment.

A SHORT HISTORY

Ozone was discovered in 1785, but it wasn't used in medicine until the late 1800s with the Florida Medical Association publishing the first medical textbook on the applications of ozone therapy.

Ozone was initially used as a disinfectant in both dental and surgical settings. In 1896, Nikola Tesla patented the first ozone generator in the United States and was the first to create ozonated olive oil.

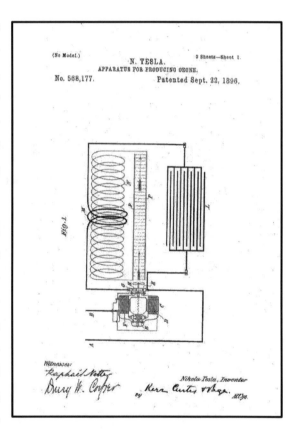

Ozone therapy developed in the early 1900s in the United States and Germany and then later in Russia and Cuba. As with many treatments, the development of antibiotics and steroids truncated research in the area of ozone therapy. In the 1970s, ozone therapy began to take off through research at the Russian State Academy of Medicine of Nizhny Novgorod. In the 1980s, Cuba adopted ozone therapy and established a research center for it.

In the twenty-first century, a concerted effort to establish ozone therapy as a scientifically based treatment has led to the increase of research at an unprecedented rate, culminating in hundreds of new studies over the past few years.[7]

INTERNATIONAL ACCEPTANCE

After I started O3Vets, I quickly saw the need to provide training for veterinarians who were interested in adding ozone therapy to their practices. So, as any logical entrepreneur with a passion for trying new things would have done, I decided to host my first training class in Tokyo . . . in Japanese. I partnered with Dr. Margo Roman and a respected Japanese veterinarian, Dr. Makoto Washizu. Without them, this would have fallen flat, but we pulled it off and put on a two-day class complete with a wet lab and simultaneous interpretation at Nippon Veterinary and Life Science University where Dr. Washizu taught. Since 2012, the number of Japanese ozone vets has continued to grow into the hundreds.

In 2019, I was introduced to Dr. Jean Joaquim who holds a number of important positions within the Brazilian veterinary community. He is also the head of the Brazilian Veterinary Ozone Therapy Organization. Dr. Joaquim informed me that there are about 1,000 veterinarians in Brazil who use ozone therapy.

This treatment is starting to grow around the world as veterinarians see the results in their patients. And it's not just the veterinary community that is starting to accept this treatment. There are over 50 ozone organizations throughout the world that conduct trainings and conferences, publish studies, create procedures, and provide a framework for the safe and effective use of ozone in the medical community. Additionally, a number of governments, including those of Italy, Spain, Greece, Portugal, Turkey, Brazil, United Arab Emirates, Oman, China, Cuba, Russia, and Ukraine, have accepted ozone therapy as a safe and effective medical treatment to varying degrees.[8]

In 2008, the Russian Ozone Therapy Association published the *Handbook of Ozone Therapy*. In 2009, the German Medical Society for the Use of Ozone in Prevention published "Guidelines for the Use of Medical Ozone." In 2010, the Spanish Association of Medical Professionals in Ozone Therapy (AEPROMO) came out with *The Madrid Declaration on Ozone Therapy*. These, along with many other scientific works, have helped provide a framework for the safe and effective use of ozone therapy. I have included a list of resources in the back of this book that will provide you with more information on ozone therapy. If you're the kind who loves research, please check it out.

Is Ozone Therapy Safe?

To accept ozone therapy as a medical treatment, you must first believe that it is safe. In their 2011 publication "Ozone Therapy: A Clinical Review," authors Elvis and Ekta say, "Ozone therapy has been utilized and heavily studied for more than a century. Its effects are proven, consistent, safe and with minimal and preventable side effects."[9] In a paper entitled "Is It True That Ozone Is Always Toxic? The End of a Dogma," Dr. Velio Bocci concludes the following:

> There are a number of good experimental studies showing that exposure by inhalation to prolonged tropospheric ozone damages the respiratory system and extrapulmonary organs. The skin, if extensively exposed, may also

contribute to the damage. The undoubtful strong reactivity of ozone has contributed to establish the dogma that ozone is always toxic, and its medical application must be proscribed. Although it is less known, judiciously practiced ozone therapy is becoming very useful either on its own or applied in combination with orthodox medicine in a broad range of pathologies. The opponents of ozone therapy base their judgment on the ozone chemistry, and physicians, without any knowledge of the problem, are often skeptical.[10]

An unbiased observer will necessarily conclude that ozone therapy is safe in both humans and animals. There are just too many studies to think otherwise. But, if we're honest, there's an element of bias that we just cannot shake. It's part of being human, and it's not necessarily bad.

My wife tells me all the time how good looking she thinks I am. She has a higher view of me than anyone else, and I think that's a good bias to have because I am her husband, and her bias toward me is born out of a loyalty that is good and noble. My wife's bias causes her to see reality from a slightly distorted perspective that turns out to be good in the end. But with medicine, our desire for a certain outcome often taints our perspective causing us to overvalue the good and undervalue the bad or vice versa. The net result is, therefore, skewed. In this book, I present ozone therapy in a good light, but I am also using evidence that is overwhelmingly positive at this point.

OZONE AND ANIMALS

In 2017, I flew out to California and visited Dr. Diana Drumm who owns and operates the Animal Healing Center. She told me a story about one of her first experiences using ozone therapy:

> What's safer than oxygen? The way that we use it here at the Animal Healing Center is very similar to an oxygen delivery system. One of my first patients, Shelby, her owner had to carry her outside to pee and poop. She was coming to me for acupuncture and other things so when I got my ozone machine, I asked my client if she would be willing to give Shelby some ozone. Ozone therapy has made the difference in this dog's life. She could walk outside to pee on her own. And that makes a difference in the owners' life because they didn't have to carry her outside anymore. Some euthanasia decisions that have to do with quality of life, it really has made a huge difference.

We have studies on ozone therapy in animals dating all the way back to the 1950s.[11] The jury is no longer out. The evidence is in, and it's overwhelming. The only way to deny ozone therapy as an important treatment for animals is to ignore the evidence. Plain and simple. If you're a veterinarian and you really want to become convinced of the safety and efficacy of ozone therapy in animals, pick up a copy of *Ozone Therapy in Veterinary Medicine* by Dr. Zullyt Rodriguez. It's full of more data than I can share, and it will provide hard evidence for the skeptic.

Dr. Margo Roman has been instrumental in fighting for ozone therapy to be a recognized treatment option. As I was writing this book, she kindly reminded me that her state, Massachusetts, actually names ozone therapy as a complementary and alternative veterinary medicine (CAVM) treatment. If you go to www.mass.gov and look up 256 CMR 2.01, you'll actually find ozone therapy listed! I put an exclamation point here because you and I should both be excited about that. It's not the end, but it's a start.

It was an average day in July 2018 when I picked up the phone and was greeted by the unexpected. "Hi, this is Jason, and I work at the Out of Africa Park here in Arizona. We are having some issues with a python here and were advised by Dr. Randy Aronson to get some ozone therapy equipment so that we can treat her here at the park." The conversation that followed between Jason and I was interesting. We discussed ozone therapy, how it worked, and how it might be applied to a python.

Reptiles, birds, mammals, amphibians—I am not aware of any animal that won't benefit from ozone therapy. Animals of all sorts and kinds, both large and small, can and should be treated with ozone.

SUMMARY

Because of overwhelming supportive evidence, it's only a matter of time before ozone therapy is accepted into mainstream veterinary medicine. With at least 14 countries having accepted ozone therapy as a legitimate treatment, the United States is behind the curve.

- The FDA's position on ozone therapy as toxic is untenable.
- Ozone therapy should be judged based on safety and efficacy as demonstrated by unbiased data and not on our understanding of the ozone layer or smog and pollution.
- Ozone is a gas that consists of three oxygen atoms sharing electrons.
- Because ozone is highly reactive, it cannot be stored and will typically break down within a few hours.
- In veterinary medicine, we measure ozone in micrograms per milliliter ($\mu g/ml$).
- There are over 50 ozone organizations throughout the world, and thousands of veterinarians using ozone to treat a variety of diseases.
- Ozone therapy can be used on amphibians, mammals, birds, reptiles, and other species.

Chapter 3

How It Works

Natural forces within us are the true healers of disease.

HIPPOCRATES

In the early days of my time in ozone therapy, I attended the Michigan Veterinary Conference as an exhibitor. At that point, my knowledge of ozone therapy was limited. I remember being approached by a veterinarian who scoffed at the idea of using ozone as a medical treatment. He took advantage of my limited knowledge and made light of the idea. I still find a large number of people who would rather scoff than learn. Since you are reading this book, it's likely that you are in the learner group.

In 2017, I put on a veterinary ozone therapy training class in Columbus, Ohio. A veterinarian by the name of Dan Ahrens had been using ozone for a while, but he wasn't satisfied with his knowledge of the topic, so he decided to attend our class. After the class, he told me the story of a patient that had been carried into his clinic:

> It's a protocol that we use on all of our cancer cases
> now.... A Golden Retriever had a diagnosis of a cardiac

cancer that had metastasized to the lungs and to the liver. She came in and we did ozone therapy with UV daily for five days and then twice the second week and then had an ultrasound done by a specialist from Texas A&M and she could find no cancer. We're six months into it now, and we're completely cancer free.

It works—for some, the fact that it works is enough. They don't need the data. Anecdotal information or the advice from a friend is sufficient. I don't fall into this camp, but my wife does. She enjoys research and learning about health—in fact, she knows a lot more than me—but she'll also become a believer when a friend or a YouTube influencer raves about their experience. We don't need to rely on a friend, a YouTube video, or anecdotal information from a trusted colleague. We already have reliable evidence of the safety and efficacy of ozone therapy, so let's dive in.

THE PROBLEM

We know that lack of oxygen at a cellular level and chronic inflammation are at the root of the problems that ozone therapy addresses. From there, it gets more complex.

The body is a never-ending synthesis of biological reactions working in unison to maintain a healthy balance. This is known as homeostasis. When a minor disturbance occurs, the body is able to compensate and overcome it. However, in the case of long-lasting disturbances that block biological regulation, homeostasis is disrupted, and chronic disease can occur.

Systems biology attempts to identify the complex interactions between biological systems and develop medicines that work synergistically with the body to heal. Even in the age of technology, understanding these complex interactions is an incredibly difficult challenge. Take, for example, the body of a dog. We understand that for life to exist in that body, it must have a musculoskeletal system that works in symphony with the cardiovascular system, which works congruently with the immune system, which works in harmony with the digestive system, which contributes to the function of the urinary system. . . . You get the point. All of our biological systems work in harmony, but if dysregulation occurs in just one of these systems, it can have a detrimental effect on many of them. The longer the dysregulation continues without being corrected, the more negative effect it has upon the body.

The specific dysregulation that occurs in many chronic illnesses is the overproduction of immune cells and the underproduction of antioxidants, which leads to oxidative stress and inflammation. This is the obvious problem, but how did we get there? As we drill into the problem of dysregulation, which leads to poor oxygen utilization and inflammation, we have uncovered something that no one at first expected.

Much of the problem boils down to lack of cellular communication.

Dysregulation is the general problem, but to understand ozone therapy we need to understand that the dysregulation comes about through compromised cellular signaling—not just cellular signaling in general, but a specific type of cellular signaling called redox signaling.

Redox signaling refers to a cellular process known as reduction-oxidation or redox. As oxidative molecules build up in a cell, a signal is transmitted all the way to the nucleus of the cell, which results in cellular repair or replacement. You can think of redox signaling molecules as the military comms for your cells. Redox signaling is the complicated messaging system responsible for sending the information necessary to maintain a healthy balance of all types of cells and keep all related processes going.

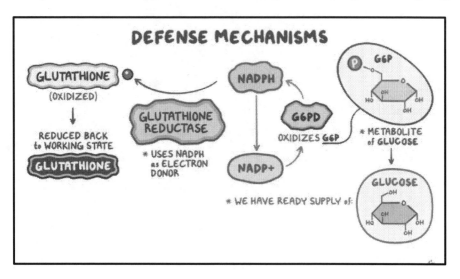

As we look more closely at redox signaling, a central molecule to maintaining proper redox signaling is glutathione. Glutathione has both an oxidized form (GSSG) and a reduced form (GSH). In healthy, resting cells, the ratio of GSH:GSSG can exceed 100:1, but in cases of oxidative stress, that ratio can be reduced to 10:1 or even as low as 1:1. Because this ratio is such a good measurement of oxidative stress, it is a commonly used indicator of total oxidative stress. When this ratio gets messed up, our comms are down, and the enemy (dysregulation) will advance and overrun our position. But the importance of GSH doesn't stop with signaling. It is considered one of the most important antioxidants, crucial to the scavenging of free radicals and detoxification of heavy metals.

In healthy cells, the reaction of glutathione and hydrogen peroxide (H_2O_2) is what initiates redox signaling. When oxidative stress is part of the picture, there are high levels of H_2O_2 in the body. But despite those high numbers, the oxidative stress inhibits H_2O_2 from carrying out its role as a redox signaling molecule.[12]

This problem is a bit more complex than researchers first thought, but all of these issues are linked. **Compromised cellular signaling leads to dysregulation, which leads to oxygen deficiency, which leads to oxidative stress and inflammation, which are linked to a variety of serious age-related diseases, including diabetes, cardiovascular, autoimmune disease, and cancer.**

OZONE AS A BIOREGULATOR

If you only take away one thing from this section, understand this: **Ozonides replace hydrogen peroxide and act as redox molecules to regulate inflammation and immune function.**

We first learned how ozone worked through studies and experiments in water treatment. Unfortunately, this understanding was translated to the medical field, which has led to the rejection of ozone as a legitimate treatment. Regulatory bodies such as the FDA mistakenly surmised that the germicidal action of ozone was the key to its efficacy as a medical treatment while completely overlooking the hormetic action of ozone as a bioregulator.

It used to be that hydrogen peroxide was considered toxic when inside the body, but more recent studies[13] show that it is crucial to immune function. As with anything, the key is balance. Too much or too little, and regulation can be blocked, which then leads to degeneration.

When using the term "redox," I'm referring to a reaction that includes reduction (red) and oxidation (ox). In their review of redox signaling, authors Forman, Ursini, and Maiorino state, "The increasing interest in looking at redox signaling, rather than oxidative stress as a focus, has given some of us chemistry-oriented biomedical scientists, the opportunity to consider this chemistry in terms of explaining how **reactive molecules can be part of normal physiology or at least not lead to pathology**." They go on to say that "only hydroperoxides clearly fit the role of a second messenger." Hydroperoxides? Yes, just keep reading.

When ozone comes into contact with the body, it reacts with numerous elements but most notably with unsaturated fatty acids, which contain double bonds. Ozone reacts with those double bonds to form ozonides. These ozonides are semi-reactive molecules that are a normal part of our physiology, and they become a secondary messenger that interacts with glutathione to initiate redox signaling.[14] To go back to our previous illustration, ozonides pick up the comms from hydrogen peroxide and call in the information to restore homeostasis to the cell.

While we are still gathering data on the interaction of ozone with various biological components, it's *likely* that ozone takes over the role of hydrogen peroxide to carry out its signaling responsibilities. This wasn't always thought to be the case. In fact, through the 1980s and 1990s, Dr. Velio Bocci's work focused on ozone's effect on red blood cell metabolism with oxygen utilization as well as the impact on immune cells with immunomodulation as the end result. It wasn't until 1998 that Leon et al. published a paper on the role of ozone in redox signaling and oxidative preconditioning.[15] We now know that the effect of ozone on the body depends on what ozone reacts with. It is also now understood that it is likely the ozonide (hydroxy hydroperoxide) that is pharmacologically active.

Contrary to the long-chain peroxides that result in chronic oxidative stress, the mild oxidative stress put on the body through the administration of ozone therapy is very different. Oxygen and OH radicals create a more permanent and destructive version of oxidative stress, often forming long-chain peroxides that are much more stable than ozonides.

There are certain markers for oxidative stress including H_2O_2, malondial-dehyde (MDA) and total hydroperoxides (TH) One seemingly small detail that makes all the difference is the fact that these oxidative markers are long-chain peroxides with a central hydroperoxide group, which gives them a long half-life and allows them to do damage when unchecked by antioxidants. These long-chain peroxides caused by oxygen and OH radicals create a perfect environment for chronic inflammatory diseases like cancer, arthritis, and various infections. Ozonides are different. Ozonides are short-chain peroxides and, although still reactive, are non-radical.

When a patient is suffering from an inflammatory condition and their oxidative stress markers are high, it would seem counterintuitive to infuse more oxidative products into their system. However, when it comes to ozone, a beautiful paradox holds true. When ozonides take the place of H_2O_2, they work as a bioregulator and initiate signal transduction through the NFkB and Nrf2 pathways when dealing with oxidative stress and inflammatory processes. We'll talk more about these two pathways shortly.

The Four Mechanisms

I'm basing the following information on various studies, but instead of referencing each sentence in this section, I have leaned heavily on two scientific articles found at PubMed.org. They are "Ozone in Medicine. The Low-Dose Ozone Concept and Its Basic Biochemical Mechanisms of Action in Chronic Inflammatory Diseases"[16] and "Ozone therapy: an overview of pharmacodynamics, current research, and clinical utility."[17]

So far, we've discovered that ozone therapy works by helping intracellular communication, but understanding that process doesn't give us a full picture of how ozone therapy works. We now need to look at the end-game of ozone therapy.

There are four common areas of research that demonstrate the multifaceted effect of ozone. The following mechanisms of action seem to be most prominent:

1. Regulation of Antioxidants
2. Regulation of Immune Cells
3. Circulation and Oxygen Uptake
4. Antimicrobial Effect

One of these factors by itself would be good. All four of them working together can be miraculous.

Mechanism 1: Regulation of Antioxidants. Life is a precious balance. Nowhere is this more evident than within the cells that make up our bodies, which are constantly self-monitoring to maintain levels of all types of cells, including immune cells, blood cells, and stem cells. Balancing the process of oxidation with antioxidants is one of the most central processes to health. Everyone knows that antioxidants are good. Grab a box of Kellogg's Smart Start® cereal and you're promised "Original Antioxidants." I'm not certain what unoriginal antioxidants are, but that investigation is beyond the scope of this book. Foods that are high in vitamins, including A, C, and E, will also be rich in antioxidants. Certain grains, berries, and nuts provide essential antioxidants. That's great. But what about what we discussed in chapter one? What about oxygen utilization?

Oxygen is also good. There must be a certain level of oxidation at all times, or our bodies will not produce the energy they need to survive. **It really is all about balance—homeostasis.** When disease attacks the body of an animal, or as age sets in, that balance is disrupted. Nowhere is that disruption felt more than in the mitochondria. The mitochondria are the powerhouse of the cell, producing the fuel (ATP) that pets need to have energy and to stay healthy. The mitochondria make up about 50% of cell weight and 10% of body weight. They are enormously important, and their function is tied directly to oxygen utilization. The importance of this statement cannot be overemphasized.

I did a quick search on PubMed and found 10,666 papers and studies that are directly or indirectly related to the link between mitochondria and aging. There were 31,269 studies related to mitochondria and disease. The link between oxygen utilization, mitochondria, aging, and disease is irrefutable.[18]

But before we fully understand the link between oxygen utilization, anti-oxidants, and ozone, I need to introduce the free radical. A free radical is a highly reactive molecule created from oxygen and is a normal and necessary part of cellular life. Reactive Oxygen Species (ROS) are a group of free radicals that play a prominent role in how ozone therapy works. Free radicals are not bad, but an overproduction of free radicals can cause serious damage and lead to deteriorated health.[19] Consequently, free radicals must be tightly controlled, and that's what leads us to the antioxidant capacity of the body. The more efficient the antioxidant system is, the less free radical damage exists and the longer our pets will live. On the other hand, as the antioxidant system depletes, free radicals go unchecked and can lead to a host of degenerative diseases, including cancer, asthma, diabetes, dementia, macular degeneration, and inflammation of joints.

As we've already learned, when ozone is administered and reacts with unsaturated fatty acids, it creates ozonides that produce a mild oxidative stress.

Another result of ozone is that it activates a pathway known as nuclear factor erythroid factor 2 (Nrf2), which helps regulate the antioxidant defenses.[20] This is a complex mechanism which is still under investigation, but there is good evidence and strong theory to support it.

Ozonides are bioregulators that work in a less aggressive way than many of the reactive oxygen species (ROS), and they reduce glutathione (GSH) to regulate antioxidants through this Nrf2 pathway. Besides signaling for the production of antioxidants, ozonides take the place of more aggressive oxidative compounds like superoxide dismutase (SOD) and catalase (CAT), performing their task in a way that decreases oxidative stress.[21]

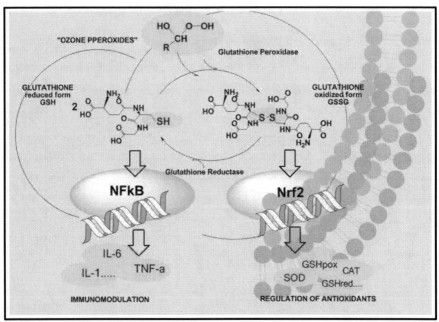

Viebahn-Haensler R, León Fernández OS. Ozone in Medicine. The Low-Dose Ozone Concept and Its Basic Biochemical Mechanisms of Action in Chronic Inflammatory Diseases. Int J Mol Sci. 2021 Jul 23;22(15):7890. doi: 10.3390/ijms22157890. PMID: 34360655; PMCID: PMC8346137

The production of these antioxidants includes glutathione, heme oxygenase-1 (HO-1), and heat shock proteins. These and other antioxidants then actively search out and neutralize the free radicals. Since ozone is an oxidant, it seems strange to many that it would have this effect on the body, which is why many studies refer to this process as "the ozone paradox."

Another part of this antioxidant puzzle is how ozone gas affects two other gases—carbon monoxide (CO) and nitric oxide (NO). (Don't confuse nitric oxide, which is important for healthy blood vessels, with nitrous oxide, which is also known as laughing gas. These are very different gases. It's important to understand that carbon monoxide in the right amounts is an essential part of a healthy body.)

As stated earlier, that can help produce heat shock proteins (HSPs). HSP32 is responsible for the formation of carbon monoxide and nitric oxide. What's becoming clear is that, through the production of HSP32, ozone helps regulate the anti-inflammatory and pro-inflammatory effects of carbon monoxide. When it comes to nitric oxide, the enzymes produced as a result of this oxidative stress are responsible for its creation. HSP70 is another heat shock protein that protects cells from inflammation, cancer, aging, and neurodegenerative disorders. This and other heat shock proteins have become the focus of numerous studies and has resulted in many pharmaceutical companies producing drugs that will upregulate them.[22]

Putting all the pieces of this complex puzzle together is a work in progress, but the role that ozone plays in producing these heat shock proteins is likely a crucial part of how it works. If veterinarians follow guidelines for the proper administration of ozone, you will not fall prey to contributing to chronic oxidative stress.

In summary, the central role that ozone therapy plays in the regulation of antioxidants seems to come through its ability to stimulate the Nrf2 pathway, thereby regulating the production of antioxidants primarily through the reduction of glutathione.[23]

Mechanism 2: Circulation and Oxygen Uptake. Ozone increases the flow of oxygen across the cell membrane, which, in turn, increases oxygen levels inside the cell. This leads to higher energy levels in the mitochondria by improving the efficiency of the respiratory chain. In red blood cells, glycolysis—the breakdown of blood sugars for cell use—is an essential process for cellular energy. An enzyme that aids in this process is called phosphofructokinase. The increase of this enzyme through application of ozone to a patient also increases cellular energy (ATP) and starts a shift in the hemoglobin that enables it to offload oxygen more easily to ischemic tissues. Besides improving oxygen deliverability, ozone also improves the flow of the blood throughout the body.

As ozone therapy is applied repeatedly—around 10 to 20 times for ischemic conditions—Lipid Oxidative Products (LOPs) are generated with enough consistency to reach the bone marrow and stimulate the production of a specially outfitted erythrocyte along with antioxidant enzymes. These "super-gifted erythrocytes" are really just carrying a larger amount of an enzyme (G6PD) that enables them to work more efficiently. For three to four months, they can powerfully improve oxygen transport and uptake throughout the body.

We know that ozone can improve blood circulation and oxygen delivery, but it can also protect the body against oxidative stress by preparing or preconditioning the cells. This effect is similar to the effect of exercise for a racehorse. The exercise will prepare him for the stress that his body will undergo during the race and allow him to thrive under that stress. This oxidative preconditioning occurs when ozone is applied to the patient and a small, controlled oxidative stress occurs. This stress leads to the formation of antioxidant enzymes, which leads to an increase in erythrocytes that have been trained to withstand oxidative stress.

Another way that ozone therapy affects blood flow and oxygen delivery is by increasing levels of nitric oxide and prostacyclin, a lipid molecule known to result in vasodilation. Vasodilation is desirable, especially when dealing with ischemic tissue, because it widens the blood vessels, leading to better blood flow and more oxygen delivery.

Mechanism 3: Immune System Activation. We've already talked about how H_2O_2 is an important element that acts as a signal to the immune system. The lack of adequate signal transduction by H_2O_2 has opened the door for ozonides to come in and do this important work, but how does it do it? To answer this question, we need to understand the role of the Nuclear Factor Kappa B (NFkB) pathway. The NFkB pathway has long been considered pro-inflammatory, and there is no question that this protein can turn the production of certain immune cells on, in particular a variety of cytokines and leukocytes. It is now becoming more apparent that the NFkB pathway also contributes to apoptosis of leukocytes as inflammation is resolved.[24] This discovery fits with the hypothesis of how ozone can work to both increase and decrease the production of various immune cells during the inflammatory phase of an illness.

As ozonides interact with GSH, NFkB is translocated to the cell nucleus, which results in protein synthesis and the release of cytokines such as IL-1, IL-2 and TNF-a. To date, there are 35 known interleukins that have been discovered. All of them are considered Cytokines. Cytokines are molecular messengers that help cells communicate. Without these messengers, the body wouldn't be able to destroy cells like bacteria, viruses, or cancer cells. The reason that ozone therapy is so good at treating infections is because it has been tied directly to its ability to stimulate the production of cytokines through the NFkB pathway. What's more, ozonides also activate growth factors which, at times, can lead to the release of even more cytokines and encourage tissue repair after an injury. Low doses of ozone can also inhibit excessive inflammation by suppressing the production of a lipid called prostaglandin and releasing a vasodilator (Bradykinin,) which lowers blood pressure and increases the release of macrophages and leukocytes—cells that are central to a properly functioning immune system.

Mechanism 4: Germicidal Activity. Most people who don't know anything about ozone therapy think that it must work by killing bacteria and viruses. I find that this widespread assumption is a roadblock to understanding and utilizing ozone therapy appropriately because it limits the true multifaceted effect of ozone on cells.

When using ozone topically, there is a direct oxidation of pathogens resulting in wound cleansing and an immediate cellular signaling to release growth factors. Ozone is profoundly more beneficial than something like hydrogen peroxide which, although it sterilizes, is cytotoxic and will actually have a negative effect on the healing process.[25]

High concentrations of ozone can be used topically because they are able to disinfect quickly and effectively. We use ozone topically through limb bagging, ozonated fluids, and ozonated oils, but using ozone gas allows for the highest concentrations. These high concentrations and larger doses are perfect as an antimicrobial when applied topically. The ability of ozone to destroy pathogens via direct contact cannot be duplicated by other substances and should be taken full advantage of within medicine. Contrary to the indirect mechanism that we see at work internally, the direct effect of ozone in external applications uses OH radicals and H_2O_2 to its advantage to reduce pathogenic load.

Another equally important effect of topical ozone is the release of the transforming growth factor beta (TGF-B), which is important when healing a wound as it speeds up the tissue remodeling phase. When growth factors are released, a number of cellular responses are affected, including the attraction of fibroblasts, which help to build the extracellular matrix. This profound stimulation of cellular proliferation, along with the immediate and prolonged antiseptic effect, is crucial to healing. It's no wonder that topical ozone can have incredible effects that go far beyond chlorhexidine or iodine.

SUMMARY

In summary, your understanding of how ozone therapy works will determine how you use it to treat animals. Because of its ability to reduce inflammation and promote cellular oxygenation, ozone therapy is a powerful veterinary tool that can help almost every patient.

- Ozone therapy addresses dysregulation of immune cells and the underproduction of antioxidants, which lead to oxidative stress and inflammation.
- The primary effect of ozone therapy applied topically is antimicrobial. It also increases growth factors to heal faster.
- The primary effect of ozone therapy applied systemically is that it acts as a bioregulator. Ozonides replace hydrogen peroxide and act as redox molecules to regulate inflammation and immune function.
- The four main mechanisms of action—antioxidant capacity, circulation and oxygen uptake, immune modulation, and germicidal activity—rely to varying degrees on redox signaling.

Chapter 4

How to Administer Ozone

Because of its incredible versatility, there is no doubt in my mind that if I were permitted only one therapy to use with my patients, ozone therapy would be the clear choice.

DR. FRANK SHALLENBERGER

I used to laugh out loud at the Geico commercials with the slogan "So easy, even a caveman could do it." The image of a caveman in the modern world disgusted with the idea that he was being disparaged is just funny.

Ozone therapy is so easy to administer that, even if you're a caveman, you'll be able to figure it out.

Dr. Marlene Siegel is an ozone therapy trainer for O3Vets. During our trainings, she never fails to mention that ozone therapy is a technician-driven treatment. What that means in a clinical setting is that, while the vet tech is treating the patient with ozone, the veterinarian is freed up to do the things that only they can do. In the home, this means that even the average pet owner will be able to master some of the ozone administration methods discussed in this chapter—and that's a good feeling.

One by one, let's look at the different administration methods that you can employ using ozone. I'll categorize them under the following headings:

- Oils
- Fluids
- Insufflations
- Injections
- Blood
- Inhalation

(One important note before we dive into these administration methods. We will not deal comprehensively in this book with each protocol. If you want a step-by-step protocol, along with the required items for each administration method, you can find that in a guide that my company, O3Vets, compiled. It's called the *Veterinary Ozone Treatment Guide*. Make sure to pick up a copy. Between that guide and this book, you'll be thoroughly prepared to practice ozone therapy for animals.)

We'll start with the most basic methods that are sometimes used in the home and then address the methods that are typically only performed in a clinic. Keep in mind that when I discuss using ozone in the home, I assume that it is under the guidance of a veterinarian. Using ozone at home is really the same concept as taking medication home to administer as directed by the veterinarian. Once you know how and when to administer ozone, it's not that complicated, however, most injections or blood-related methods will need to be done in a veterinary clinic.

OILS

I can't think of an easier way to apply ozone than to rub it into the skin. It's easy, fast, and efficient. But let me back up and tell you how ozone oil works. In the introduction to "Ozone Therapy in Veterinary Medicine," Dr. Silvia Menendez explains it this way:

> The different actions of ozonized oils on the different diseases of the integumentary system [the outer layer of a body] are another of the most relevant issues. Among these, its broad-spectrum germicidal, anti-inflammatory, healing and stimulating action of antioxidant systems are highlighted making it a drug of choice for the treatment of a wide range of dermatological diseases.

How it works. Ozone has a very short half-life. It degrades very quickly in air and fluids, but this isn't true of ozonated oils. When an oil is ozonated, it has a shelf life of over two years.

Many different types of vegetable oils can be infused with ozone (ozonated) and then be used therapeutically. The most common types of ozonated oil include olive, sunflower, and coconut.

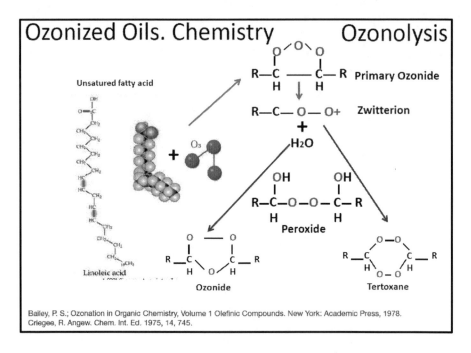

Bailey, P. S.; Ozonation in Organic Chemistry, Volume 1 Olefinic Compounds. New York: Academic Press, 1978.
Criegee, R. Angew. Chem. Int. Ed. 1975, 14, 745.

Vegetable oils contain unsaturated fatty acids, which, in turn, contain a carbon atom linked to another carbon atom through a double bond. A double bond means that these two carbon atoms share four electrons instead of two, and their double bond makes the connection between the two atoms stronger. As these double bonds come into contact with ozone, they are oxidized and disappear. If an oil has a higher level of double bonds, that oil can hold more ozone. Therefore, some oils are considered stronger than others.

An important side note here is that just because an oil is more potent doesn't mean that it's more effective. There is no evidence that would suggest that oils of greater strength work better than those of lesser strength. Although companies will market a variety of oils, don't worry so much about what type of oil you should use. Just make sure that you are purchasing through a reputable company that knows its product (like O3Vets).[26]

The most common way to measure the level of ozone in an oil is through the peroxide value. This value measures the peroxides in the oil. Generally, the longer an oil is ozonated, the more peroxides it will have and the thicker it will become. The type of oil also determines the amount of ozone that it can hold. For example, coconut oil is a naturally low-strength oil; olive is a medium-strength oil, and sunflower seed is a high-strength oil.[27]

It may seem like the process to ozonate an oil is simple, but I would never recommend doing it at home or in the clinic for two reasons.

Firstly, as oil is ozonated, its temperature increases. Without the proper equipment, the ability to protect against fire hazard is reduced. I have personally talked with an ozone expert who sells ozone oils for a living. In the early days, he blew up his garage while making ozone oils.

Secondly, without the proper equipment and process in place, unwanted products such as formaldehyde are created in the oil which can negatively impact the patient.[28]

It's not uncommon to see or hear of someone who ozonates their own oils. They will connect an ozone generator to an oxygen source and run the ozone into a glass flask that contains the oil they would like to ozonate. As the ozone bubbles into the oil, the oil absorbs the ozone. The left-over oxygen then escapes through an exhaust port connected to a destruct, which scavenges any ozone that remains so that it doesn't escape into the air to be breathed. Depending on a number of factors, including the concentration and volume of the ozone, the amount of oil, the temperature of the oil, and the presence of water as a catalyst, the ozonation time can take anywhere from four hours to a week. The problem is that the user has unknowingly created by-products that will remain in the oil and may be an irritant to the skin.[29]

What oils treat. Although oils are most commonly used to treat skin conditions, they can also be used orally or rectally in the form of a suppository. Some of the specific conditions treated with ozonated oil are:

- Skin infections
- Surgery Sites
- Gingivitis
- Ulcers
- Wounds
- Hot spots

How to administer oils. Oils are the simplest method to administer. Simply apply the oil to the affected area one to three times daily or as directed by a veterinarian. There is no exact dosing needed, but it should be applied across the entire area if possible. Products like Hydrogel 15% from Honest O3 can be rubbed into the gums and tongue to treat oral conditions. Another product from Honest O3, Pet Liniment 10%, is an easy-to-use formula that absorbs more quickly than standard ozone oils. These products are not only more user-friendly, but they also have a more pleasant odor than traditional ozone oils because of how they are manufactured.[30]

It's possible that ozone oils may irritate the skin in certain patients. If this happens, you may try using a different type of oil to see if the issue was the ozone itself or the type of oil used. If irritation persists, you should use a different ozone administration method.

Tips for using oils:

- Don't attempt to make your own ozone oils.
- Ozone creams and gels are more user-friendly and less pungent than oils.

- Oils are typically applied two times per day but can be used more frequently.[31]
- Moist dermatitis may need to be treated using ozonated saline instead of ozone oils to avoid excess trapped moisture.

FLUIDS

Ozone gas will dissolve into various fluids. This is especially useful because fluids can be used all over the body. In my opinion, the most important accessory for the veterinarian is the fluid bubbler. Everyone should know how to use a fluid bubbler and take full advantage of this method of administration.

How it works. Bubbling fluids is almost exactly the same as the process of bubbling ozone into oil. A tank with medical-grade oxygen feeds the ozone generator, which is connected to a fluid bubbler. The ozone gas is piped down a slender tube in the middle of the bubbler that terminates in a diffuser stone. The diffuser stone is slightly more effective than a single hole at the end of the tube. The purpose of the diffuser stone is to create hundreds of tiny bubbles that travel through the fluid. Since hundreds of small bubbles have more surface area than a few large bubbles, these bubbles quickly ozonate the fluid. In contrast, the oil bubbler doesn't need a diffuser stone because the purpose of using a diffuser stone is not to ozonate the oil quickly but to create ozonides. Connected to the fluid bubbler is a secondary exhaust tube that runs to a destruct. In this setup, it's very important to have a destruct to neutralize any excess ozone that is not absorbed into the fluid so that it is not released into the air and breathed by the patient or user.

Saline and distilled water. Let's start this section by noting that there has been a lot of controversy over the use of ozonated saline when infused intravenously. In chapters three and six of his book entitled *Ozone. A New Medical Drug,* Dr. Velio Bocci discusses at length the concept of ozonating both distilled water and saline. He concludes that, "I must strongly recommend to avoid the use of ozonated saline owing to inherent toxicity or/and doubtful pharmacologic activity."

The World Federation of Ozone Therapy produced a signed statement in 2017 that presented ozonated saline as inducing "the generation of dangerous oxidized chlorine derivatives" and having been shown "to induce mutagenicity and toxicity in clinical reports." Even the authors of the Madrid Declaration on Ozone Therapy jumped on the bandwagon in the early years.[32] It wasn't that they thought saline was always a bad idea since there was no talk of external use being a problem, but the real concern was if ozonated saline was to be infused intravenously.

The camp that refused intravenous saline as an option was not alone. There was an equally adamant group of scientists and doctors who approved the use of intravenous saline and set out to prove that it was not only effective but also safe. In 2020, a variety of papers were published both for and against the use of IV ozonated saline. Among them was a study from China that was less than definitive but seemed to suggest that ozonated saline contains chlorate and that, if the saline is prepared in a plastic container, the reaction of the ozone with the plastic may increase the chlorate content. Their conclusion in this study was that we don't really know if the levels of chlorate are safe for intravenous infusion, although there are studies which seem to indicate they are.

Another of those studies was produced in the same year and came from Italy.[33] In this study, Dr. Gregorio Martinez notes that there are numerous recent studies that utilized ozonated saline solution (O_3SS) as a novel treatment for COVID-19. Dr. Martinez states that "studies using O_3SS are increasingly being disseminated in scientific databases and the retrograde arguments that qualify it from 'placebo' to 'tumor-generating' are being left behind." That being said, the concern of a number of scientists in both camps is that ozonating saline at concentrations over 8 μg/ml may lead to the formation of chlorates or hypochlorites that could be cytotoxic. Because of this, ozonated saline that is infused intravenously should be ozonated at a concentration below 8 μg/ml, while ozonated saline used topically can be ozonated at higher concentrations.

The two fluids that I recommend for use are 0.9% sodium chloride (normal saline) and distilled or bi-distilled water. Bi-distilled water is ultra-pure and will absorb and hold ozone for significantly longer than regular distilled water. However, the cost and availability of bi-distilled water prohibit it from becoming a viable option for most. On the other hand, distilled water is readily available at almost every grocery store. I'm asked all the time about using tap water, or various types of purified water. The answer is that, yes, you can, but the level of ozone absorption into these fluids will be significantly less, and the ozone that is absorbed will break down quicker as the ozone reacts with impurities and minerals.

Normal saline is something that every veterinarian has on hand and uses frequently. Normal saline that has been ozonated is something that every veterinarian *should* have on hand and will come to love once they see the remarkable benefits. Unlike water, saline mimics body fluids and can safely be infused into an animal's body either subcutaneously or intravenously. There are other fluids like Lactated Ringers Solution (LRS) and Normosol®, which are commonly used in the place of saline, but I do not recommend ozonating these fluids as the ozone may react with some of the components and, over time, create a film on the inside of the glass bubbler.

A common misconception is that if you ozonate a fluid at a high concentration (i.e., 70 ug/ml), you will get a fluid with a similar concentration. The reality is that, with a pure fluid such as 0.9% Sodium Chloride (normal saline) or distilled water, the concentration of ozone will top out at 10-25% of the concentration used to ozonate the fluid. That's the upper limit of ozone that a fluid can hold. For example, if you ozonate a fluid using a gas concentration of 50 µg/ml, you'll reach a peak concentration from 5-12 µg/ml. Once fully ozonated, a fluid will also lose the ozone fairly quickly. The half-life of ozone in a sterile fluid at 70° F is approximately 45 minutes. Again, this will vary based on the type of fluid, the temperature of the fluid, and the container that it's in. Bi-distilled water will last longer than distilled water, and distilled water will last longer than saline.[34]

What it treats. The method that you use to administer the fluid will sometimes determine what you are treating. For example, eye drops will be used for conditions of the eye. Subcutaneous saline is often used as a systemic way to easily get ozone into the tissue, but it can also be injected locally around a tumor or infection. Lavaging is most often used to clean and disinfect areas that are infected or could become infected. Drinking ozonated fluids is more common in humans who have a respiratory condition or are simply suffering from the common cold. Finally, intravenous saline is used to treat systemic conditions regardless of pathology.

I'll share a little more on what is treated under each administration method below.

How to administer. Fluids are one of the most important methods to administer ozone because they can be used in so many different ways. Because of this, administering fluid will take on various forms. There isn't just one protocol, but precision with dosing and protocol for administration are not all that crucial. Here's a list of some of the ways you can use fluids for a patient.

Lavaging (Rinsing)—Externally, lavaging can be used to flush a wound, bathe a hot spot, clean an infected area, or speed the healing of a surgical site. You may use any amount from a few milliliters, in the case of a small rodent, to an entire liter or more in treating a horse. Internally, ozonated saline can be used to lavage a cavity or an organ during surgery. You may use up to a couple of liters of fluid when lavaging the uterus of a cow, but as few as ten milliliters when treating a cat.

Saline Eye Drops—These drops are often used for infections, macular degeneration, or other conditions of the eye. Once the saline is ozonated, it's really just a matter of rinsing the eye for 5-15 seconds. You can administer the eye drops via a syringe or whatever is handy to help you get the fluid into the eye.

Subcutaneous Saline—In Russia, ozonated saline has been used for many years in human medicine, but always intravenously. It should be noted that the accepted Russian protocol is to use a low concentration of ozone to ozonate the saline and simultaneously bubble the ozone into the saline while the infusion into the patient is taking place. (This differs from the generally accepted practice of subcutaneous saline for animals.) This method has been employed because it's inexpensive, effective, and easy. Often, the patient benefits from added hydration, and the ozone in the saline is easily absorbed into the bloodstream and surrounding tissue.

To administer ozonated subcutaneous saline to an animal, you'll first need to ozonate the fluid following the instructions earlier in this chapter. The next step will depend on the fluid bubbler that you have because not all bubblers are created equal. O3Vets has a 1,500 ml bubbler and a 500 ml bubbler. The larger bubbler is used in veterinary practices while the smaller one is used for home treatments. I recommend starting with one milliliter per pound of body weight. For example, if you have a 50 lb. dog, administer 50 milliliters of ozonated fluid.

Once the animal has had a few treatments, some veterinarians will use up to 150 ml of saline. If using the vet bubbler, you can run saline directly from the bubbler to the patient via an IV line with a connected needle. Opening the clamp will allow gravity to feed fluid subcutaneously. Using the 500 ml bubbler requires that you draw the fluid into a syringe before injecting it under the skin.

This simple process can be followed for many conditions including the following:

- Injections along both sides of the spine to treat degenerative disk disease or pain
- Injections into one location for systemic conditions or general wellness
- Injections around tumors
- Mange and other skin conditions

One final but important note is to be aware of any restriction that the animal has on sodium. For example, if they have kidney or blood pressure issues, it would be wise to use a different method of administration that doesn't require saline.

Drinking Water–Drinking ozonated water is much more common for human consumption than animals because animals tend to dislike the taste, but I have known pet owners who mix it with something to get their pet to drink it. This is one area where lack of scientific information makes it difficult to give suggestions. I won't pretend to be an expert on this but leave the drinking of ozonated water up to your own judgment.

Intravenous Saline—Again, this is more widely practiced in human medicine, but it can be a good way to treat systemically.

There are two camps regarding this application. One says to fully saturate the fluid (about 20–30 μg/ml,) and the other says to give fluid that has been ozonated with a low concentration of ozone (2-7 μg/ml). I cannot make a conclusive statement one way or the other. However, since the available scientific information is based on the lower concentration, you would do well to follow those guidelines and introduce a weaker concentration of ozonated fluid intravenously. Ozonated saline can be run directly from the vet bubbler if you have it, or it can be drawn up into a syringe and infused through a needle into the vein.

Each of these methods can be used to treat a variety of conditions, so don't consider my list of conditions exhaustive. This list will provide an idea of how ozonated fluids can be used.

Tips for using fluids:

- Putting the fluid bubbler on an IV pole is a more efficient way of using ozonated saline in a clinic.
- Refresh your fluid with ozone before you use it if it has sat for more than 40 minutes.
- Bubbling ozone through a fluid that has been sitting in the bubbler for days will sterilize it.
- If you send ozonated fluids back home with your clients, make sure the fluid is in a glass container with a Teflon top. Also, make sure that they refrigerate it.

- Heating the fluid will cause the ozone to break down, but the colder the fluid, the more ozone it can hold.

INSUFFLATIONS

As you look at the list of ways that ozone therapy can be administered, you may feel a little overwhelmed. How do you know which method to use? Do you need to utilize all of them? Will the treatment be as effective if the wrong method is used?

I want to remind you that just one ozone administration method is sufficient in the beginning. And sometimes, one administration method is sufficient all the way through treatment. For example, the pet owner may only use rectal insufflation and not need to deviate from it. So, if you feel a little anxiety when you see all the administration methods mentioned in this chapter, take a step back and recognize that learning and implementing these will take some time, but learning and implementing just one method is much better than not using ozone at all.

Let's now turn to insufflations. To insufflate with ozone is to blow it into a cavity of the body. We can perform insufflations into the ear, the rectum, the bladder, the teat canal of the mammary gland, or the vagina.

How it works. This method is simple and minimally invasive. To apply, draw up ozone from the generator and put it into the patient with the appropriate accessory. Similar to the previous methods, there are no needles or blood required, which makes insufflations painless and well tolerated.

What it treats. The area insufflated will determine what is being treated, but there are a few caveats. Rectal insufflation is very easy and has shown to be effective for a variety of chronic conditions. Because of this, it has become a common administration method, not only for colon conditions, but also for just about anything ozone therapy is used for. Ear insufflation can be used to treat not only the ear but head and neck conditions as well. Intramammary insufflation is primarily used on cows to treat mastitis. Although vaginal insufflation is not commonly used in animals, it is most often used to treat vaginal conditions.

How to administer. The protocol will depend upon the area you're insufflating, but for vaginal, ear, and intramammary insufflation, the applicator is connected directly to the ozone generator, and a continuous flow of ozone is infused into the cavity. Rectal insufflation is different. With this method, ozone is drawn up into a syringe or insufflation bag and infused into the colon.

Let's look at each of these individually.

Rectal Insufflation—Because ozone therapy has become standard practice in Cuban medicine, and rectal insufflation is one of the easiest administration methods, a protocol has been developed that has quite a bit of scientific backing. Rectal insufflation is administered five days a week for three weeks. The fourth week has no treatments. This cycle of three weeks on and one week off can be repeated. The Madrid Declaration on Ozone Therapy recommends repeating every 3-4 months.

In animals, I recommend a concentration of 35 µg/ml and a volume of 1 ml per pound of patient body weight (e.g., 50 ml for a 50 lb. dog). This volume can be increased as recommended by a veterinarian. To treat the patient, the ozone is drawn up into a syringe or bag, an ozone-resistant rectal catheter is connected, the tip is lubricated, and the catheter is inserted approximately three inches into the colon. The ozone is then infused, the catheter removed, and the tail (if available) is held between the legs for 30 seconds to ensure that no ozone gas passes from the colon before absorption.

Ear Insufflation—There are a couple of ways to administer ozone into the ears. The first is to use ear insufflation cups that are connected directly to the ozone generator. Ozone gas is then infused slowly into the ear canal. The challenge with this method is that it is nearly impossible to contain all the ozone without some of it escaping into the air exposing the patient and/or user to the risk of breathing in ozone gas. Because of this, it is necessary to administer this treatment in a well-ventilated area with an exhaust fan drawing any excess ozone outside. A second option is to connect an oil bubbler between the ozone generator and the ear cups so that the ozone is first bubbled through oil. This transforms the gas into ozonides and peroxides, which can then be safely breathed. You can see a demo of this method here: www.youtube.com/o3vets.

I prefer to do ear insufflation without the oil bubbler because bubbling it through oil reduces the potency of the treatment. If you do need to use the oil bubbler, increase the flow rate to ¼ LPM and the concentration to 60 µg/ml if your generator allows. If you don't have those settings, try to strike a good balance between concentration and flow rate. You can also fill a syringe with ozone and then wrap the ear with a moist hand towel to keep the ozone in as you slowly infuse 20–40 ml of a high concentration of ozone gas.

Vaginal Insufflation—Currently, there is no animal-specific applicator that makes vaginal insufflation easy. In human medicine, a special vaginal insert is available that seals the vaginal opening and provides an exhaust that runs through an ozone destruct. This protects the patient from breathing any ozone gas that escapes from the vagina. This special applicator also allows the user to hook up the ozone generator directly and run a continuous flow of ozone into the vagina for a period of 10-20 minutes at a very slow flow rate. With animals, you must draw up a syringe of ozone and slowly infuse it into the vaginal cavity using a rectal catheter. Use the same dose as you would for rectal insufflation, but infusion into the vagina should be done slower so that the ozone has more time to absorb.

Intramammary Insufflation–I am only aware of its use in cows and goats, but intramammary insufflation could be used for many species. Frankly, I'm shocked that this treatment hasn't taken off to treat mastitis on a large-scale level. One day, it will.

In a study entitled "Intramammary application of ozone therapy to acute clinical mastitis in dairy cows," Ogata and Nagahata note that "sixty percent (9/15) of cows with acute clinical mastitis treated with ozone therapy did not require any antibiotics for recovery. This newly developed ozone therapy method was proven to be effective, safe, and cost effective, and carries no risk of drug residues in milk."

Using ozone therapy as a substitute for antibiotics could collectively save dairy farmers millions of dollars in milk that would otherwise be wasted due to drug residue. It could also revolutionize the way of handling mastitis or other infectious diseases on organic farms and lead to incredible cost savings for the farmer.

The protocol is simple. An ozone generator is set up in a location near the cow, and a long silicone tube is connected from the ozone outlet on the generator to a cannula that is inserted directly into the infected teat. A concentration of 60 μg/ml is infused into the teat at 1/2 LPM for one minute. That's all there is to it. This can be done on all infected quarters and then repeated as necessary each day for a week. Alternatively, an insufflation bag with ozone can be filled and then infused into the teat instead of flowing ozone directly from the generator. This application will allow more mobility and an easier treatment.

Tips for insufflations:

- If possible, milk the cow before intramammary insufflation and perform rectal insufflation after a bowel movement. This way, more of the ozone will be absorbed into the tissue.
- Lubricating the tip of the catheter before rectal insufflation will make insertion easier.
- If you are using an oil bubbler for ear insufflation, organic olive oil is a good choice. Before using the oil for the first time, run ozone into it for two hours to help saturate the oil with ozone before use. This will ensure an effective treatment.
- Oil can be reused, but I recommend replacing it each month with fresh oil.

INJECTIONS

In this section we're going to talk exclusively about intraperitoneal injections and general injections. Although Prolo+Ozone and Ozone+Acupuncture are considered injections, I'm going to deal with those in the next chapter because they are combination treatments that add something in addition to the ozone. Also, subcutaneous saline and minor autohemotherapy (mAHT) could go into this category, but I have chosen to include those under the categories of fluids and blood, respectively.

The two injections that will be discussed use ozone gas without any additive or carrier to assist in delivery. These injections are exclusively the work of a trained veterinarian and should not be done at home.

How it works. Just as in some of the other methods, the injected ozone is absorbed into the tissue. This is especially helpful if there is a localized problem and specific goals for the problem. For example, you may want to slow the growth of a tumor. With an infection, the goal is to control and eliminate it. Veterinarians understand that the local expression is usually symptomatic of a more systemic issue, so it can be wise to combine these local injections with a systemic method as well. For example, when doing an injection of ozone around a tumor, you may also want to administer rectal insufflation. It's not always necessary, but doing a combo treatment like this can add some benefit to the treatment. You should also consider the combination of ozone and ultraviolet light (O3UV) as an even more powerful way to treat systemically. I'll talk more about this in the next chapter.

What it treats. Ozone injections usually treat a local issue. Intraperitoneal injections are typically reserved for abdominal conditions. General injections will be used to treat all the following:

- Degenerative discs
- Arthritis
- Joint injuries and pain
- Tumors
- Surgical sites
- Periodontal disease

The list could go on, but this gives a broad summary of the more common conditions treated with ozone injections. As I provide guidance, remember that there's always more than one way to administer ozone for a specific condition and that ozone therapy will benefit the patient regardless of the way it's administered. That being said, there can be more or less effective administration methods depending on the condition. I also believe that injections will often provide more benefit when you combine them with another treatment. As an example, using prolotherapy and ozone together for joints or degenerative conditions is more powerful than ozone alone.

How to administer. Injecting ozone is simple, but a good understanding of anatomy and some experience doing injections into these areas is crucial for those that will go into a joint or near an organ. The simple part is drawing up the ozone from your generator and connecting a needle to the syringe. You're now ready to do the injection. Placing the needle is the important and more difficult challenge. For joint or intraperitoneal injections, you may need to sedate the patient. I find that it's more common to sedate than not, but there are patients who tolerate these injections well without sedation. Part of the decision to sedate depends on your skill and experience. It also depends on whether you're including the prolo solution, which uses a pain-inhibiting drug called Procaine. Intra-articular injections can and should be done with precision and an understanding of exactly where you want to place the needle, but for those who are less experienced, the injections may be done around a joint instead.

General Injections—Most often, general injections are reserved for injecting into or around a tumor but may also include injections into the mouth or surgical site. Injections into or around a tumor are quick and can be done without sedation. Simply draw up the desired amount of ozone at a concentration of 15-20 µg/ml and inject it into one to three locations around the tumor or directly into the tumor. The volume injected will vary depending on the size of the animal. A cat or small dog will commonly get 2-5 ml while a horse will get 10-20ml. Injections into surgical sites may be done in much the same way.

For injections into the mouth, a smaller amount (.5-1 ml) is used at the same concentration and injected under the gums or into an area of concern. This should be done while the patient is under sedation.

Intraperitoneal Injections–In laboratory studies, intraperitoneal injections have been done for quite some time. However, in the veterinary clinic, they haven't been as common. I have found a number of veterinarians who have utilized this particular method, and it can be an effective way to administer ozone. The benefit is that gaseous ozone is delivered directly into the peritoneum and is absorbed into the tissue. The downside to this method is that, for less experienced or more cautious veterinarians, it can require sedation and ultrasound guidance to ensure safety.

In her book *Ozone Therapy in Veterinary Medicine*, Dr. Zullyt Zamora Rodriguez mentions that these injections have been successfully used for canine oncological diseases, specifically of the head and neck, though she doesn't go into detail. This method is usually administered via a butterfly needle attached to an ozone syringe while the animal is under anesthesia. The ozone is infused into the peritoneum under ultrasound guidance to ensure safety. The dose is commonly 2-3 ml of ozone per pound of body weight at 50 µg/ml.

Tips for injections:

- Lower concentrations will sting less. If pain is an issue, consider lowering the concentration of the ozone.
- Intraperitoneal injections may need to be done under ultrasound guidance.

IN THE BLOOD

There are three common administration methods that involve the use of the patient's blood. They are:

- Major Autohemotherapy (MAHT)
- Minor Autohemotherapy (mAHT)
- Direct Intravenous (DIV)

While both MAHT and mAHT have a good history of use within veterinary and human medicine, the third method that we will discuss in this section has had its share of controversy. A technique for injecting ozone directly into the vein developed alongside the evolution of ozone therapy. This is called DIV ozone. This technique is inexpensive, easy, and fast. However, the idea of injecting gas into a vein is contrary to conventional wisdom. It may come as no surprise that DIV has been rejected as a valid administration method by several human medical ozone organizations throughout Europe. On one side, practitioners in human medicine are doing this daily and say that it is safe and effective. On the other side, organizations tasked with preserving the image and safety of the treatment reject it and strongly oppose its use.

As we have already seen ozone therapy is a safe treatment. There have been so few adverse events that there are almost no negative reports available. The few deaths that have occurred have been in humans due to embolism as the result of the misuse of this administration method. An embolism is an obstruction in the artery that can cause serious injury or death. In this case, an air bubble causes the obstruction.

So, here's the question: Should DIV be a legitimate method of administration for animals?

The answer is yes and no. Let me explain. Every veterinarian and medical doctor have been taught that they shouldn't inject oxygen into a vein because it could cause an embolism. At a certain point, that's true, but how much oxygen does it take to create this dreaded condition? Well, the smaller the patient, the less blood volume they have and the more likely an embolism. So, for a Yorkie, the risk is significantly higher than for a Mastiff. However, for the cow or horse, the risk is reduced so much that it becomes an incredibly safe treatment.

I've personally talked to two veterinarians who, because of circumstances, had to put a cow down. As an experiment, they pumped oxygen into the vein of the cow as quickly as possible for an extended period with no ill effect to the cow. One used syringes of oxygen, and the other used an air pump. I'm not advocating for you to try this, but these experiments illustrate just how much oxygen can be tolerated by a large animal. While I would never recommend using DIV in human medicine or on small animals, I do believe that there is a place for it in the treatment of large animals.

Dr. Judith Shoemaker is a wonderful example of a veterinarian who has used this administration method on horses for over 20 years with excellent results. In a webinar I did with Dr. Shoemaker, she had this to say:

> I have administered tens of thousands of DIV ozone treatments to horses, and I'm very comfortable with the technique that I use. I will tell you, next to being a veterinarian and doing chiropractic and acupuncture, which is my stock and trade, having an ozone generator has done more good for more animals than any other therapy that I use. I absolutely think that this is what everybody should be doing. In fact, back in the dark ages when I went to school,

we had a live surgery pony. When we finished our surgery and had to euthanize the pony, we tried to find out how much air it would take to emboli a horse. Well, it takes about 3 liters of air infused very quickly with a pump to embolize a small pony.

Dr. Shoemaker isn't the only veterinarian I've heard this from. I remember talking with a dairy vet who told me that he once attempted to euthanize a cow by pumping air into its vein, and after about six liters, he gave up. My point here is not that we should pump air into veins but that by using the proper technique and the right equipment, ozone therapy administered intravenously to a large animal can be safe and effective.

How it works. DIV and MAHT are identical in how they work and what they treat. The only difference between these two treatments is that, with DIV, the ozone is infused into the blood while it's circulating through the body. With MAHT, the blood is removed from the body and then mixed with ozone before being reinfused into the vein. Since these administration methods are so similar, either one can be used interchangeably, providing that you are treating a large animal.

So why choose DIV over MAHT if it's more controversial? The reason has to do with how fast and easy it is to do a DIV treatment, not to mention the use of an anticoagulant can be eliminated. This makes DIV a great option for large animals.

At first glance, it would seem that MAHT is more similar to mAHT just because their names are almost identical, but these two administration methods are unique because of the amount of blood used and the location for reinjection. MAHT is injected into the vein while mAHT is injected into the muscle. I always tell people to view mAHT as an auto-vaccine that stimulates the immune system.

What it treats. Along with rectal insufflation, MAHT is the most common method of administration and is used to treat systemic conditions for both humans and animals. It should be an important and central administration method in any clinic, especially for those who also use Ultraviolet Blood Irradiation because they can be combined so easily, and together they create a powerful combination treatment.

Because DIV is used to treat the same conditions as MAHT (but just in large animals), I'm going to lump the two of them together. So what are they used to treat? Well, if we move categorically, we can cover all the major systems and diseases. They are used to treat a wide range of conditions, including cancer, autoimmune conditions, circulatory conditions, diabetes, infections, and more. But I want to get a little more specific than that. In *Ozone Therapy in Veterinary Medicine*, Dr. Zullyt Zamora Rodriguez identifies the following as ideal conditions to treat with MAHT:

- Parvovirus
- Leptospirosis
- Viral Hepatitis
- Distemper
- Hemoparasitosis

I would add several other conditions to that list for rectal insufflation that could also fall under those identified above, including:

- Chronic nephropathies
- Liver diseases
- Immune-mediated diseases
- Postoperative healing
- Arthritis
- Infections

- Lyme Disease
- Cancer

Ozone therapy needs to be habitually used to treat underlying causes in a variety of diseases, but it is NOT a silver bullet. It won't always work, and it shouldn't be a last-ditch effort to save a pet. Don't put too much faith in any one treatment but do realize that this particular treatment should be a vital piece of the puzzle for your practice or your pet.

So how should minor Autohemotherapy (mAHT) be used? According to the *Madrid Declaration on Ozone Therapy*, mAHT "is an immune stimulant therapy, comparable to auto-vaccination." They recommend that it be used for any skin conditions and allergies, and as an adjuvant for cancer and chronic debilitating pathologies. I would add that it's rare for mAHT to be done by itself. I recommend that, when possible, both MAHT and mAHt be performed together. This gives the patient a more powerful treatment and approaches the underlying conditions from two separate angles. One of the benefits of doing them together is that it takes little time to add mAHT to the end of a MAHT treatment since we already have ozonated blood.

How to administer. *MAHT*–To perform MAHT, you withdraw blood, mix it with ozone, and then infuse it back into the vein. I could leave it at that, but I'll add a little more color to this process.

First, you'll probably want to add a small amount of anticoagulant to the syringe prior to drawing the blood—50 units of heparin per 1 ml of blood should be sufficient. Draw up 2-4 ml of blood per 10 pounds of body weight into this syringe, which we will label the "blood syringe." Next, draw up twice as much ozone at approximately 40 µg/ml. So, for example, if we have a 50-lb. dog, we'll draw 10-20 ml of blood and infuse 20-40 ml of ozone into that blood. Then, we connect the ozone syringe to the blood syringe using a female-to-female luer-lock connector and simply infuse the ozone into the blood. Once combined, you can connect a needle to the blood syringe (which now contains ozone as well) and gently rock it to mix. Next, express the oxygen from the syringe so all that's left is the ozonated blood. (Keep in mind that the ozone has all been absorbed into the blood and is no longer in gas form.) Finally, infuse the ozonated blood into the vein using the catheter already placed or a butterfly needle if you prefer. It's also wise to connect a blood filter to the needle to filter out any potential blood clots. That completes the process.

DIV–DIV ozone administration should only be used by trained professionals. Mistakenly injecting into the carotid artery instead of the jugular vein could result in serious injury or death. If you are a trained professional, following is a standard protocol that you can use.

Draw up ozone at 35 µg/ml into a syringe. Place a 25 g needle into the jugular vein and attach an extension tube. Tape the extension tube to the neck area to ensure that the needle doesn't pull out. Connect the ozone syringe and *SLOWLY* infuse it into the jugular vein. A normal dose requires 240-360 ml of ozone at 35 µg/ml, which is a total of four to six 60cc syringes. Stripping the vein with your hand and listening for a gurgling sound as the small ozone bubbles enter the bloodstream are good practices to ensure proper treatment. **Again, do not attempt to administer DIV ozone unless you are a trained professional**. Reading this book does not make you a trained professional. O3Vets has a variety of training options to help convert you into a trained professional. Visit www.o3vets.com to find out what is currently offered.

mAHT–mAHT can be used on its own, especially where drawing larger quantities of blood isn't easy, but I typically recommend doing MAHT and mAHT at the same time. It makes sense to use the last bit of blood from MAHT to perform a mAHT treatment and give the treatment that extra boost. To administer mAHT, withdraw approximately .5 ml per 20 lbs. of patient body weight and mix it with 1 ml of ozone at 35 µg/ml. This makes a 2:1 ozone-to-blood ratio. Once ozonated, shake the syringe vigorously for about 20 seconds. This will rupture blood cells and create a serum that will induce an immune response in the patient. Now inject the blood into the muscle. It can be injected in specific locations if we're treating something locally or just into the hind leg if the condition is systemic.

Tips for using ozone with blood:

- Start at the minimum recommended dose when treating an animal for the first time and then work toward the maximum recommended dose over three to four treatments.
- The *Madrid Declaration on Ozone Therapy* says that, when treating ischemic conditions with MAHT, it can take ten or more treatments to reach the point where ozone therapy helps stimulate the production of stem cells in the bone marrow. As a general rule, keep in mind that you may not see results after the first few treatments.
- Use whatever type of anticoagulant you believe works best.
- Using female to female luer-lock connectors is a better, cheaper, and more secure way to transfer the ozone from its syringe into the blood syringe.

INHALATION (NEBULIZATION)

Don't inhale ozone gas. As you learned earlier, breathing in significant quantities of ozone will eventually damage the lung lining and can lead to significant health concerns. Here the term "inhalation" refers to the inhalation of a vapor that is comprised of ozonides and peroxides and *not* ozone in its gaseous form. I should also mention that there isn't much scientific literature available for using ozone this way, although one study discusses the inhalation method to treat COVID-19.[35]

How it works. Ozone gas is bubbled into oil in a glass flask. As the ozone is forced into the bottom of the flask, little ozone bubbles make their way through the oil and eventually burst out onto the surface of the oil. At that point, the oil has absorbed the ozone and converted it into ozonides and peroxides. As the ozone continues to saturate the oil, the oxygen layer above the oil begins to fill with these elements, which are then forced out of the exhaust tube in the top of the bubbler and carried into the applicator where the patient breathes them in.

The effect that the oil has in transforming the ozone gas into ozonides and peroxides is exactly the same as when ozone is introduced into blood or tissue through rectal insufflation, MAHT, and other methods. The difference is that the chemical energy is not used up by the oil but is stored for future use. You may wonder whether the oil traps all these components instead of releasing some into the top part of the bubbler where they are forced into the patient. This doesn't happen unless you use the wrong type of oil or allow the oil to become too thick. You'll need to replace the oil eventually because it will become thick and stop serving its purpose over time.

What it treats. Inhalation of ozone most commonly treats respiratory conditions. Because there are so many other ways to administer ozone therapy, and because the potency of the ozone gas is diminished through the bubbling process, inhalation has not become a popular method, but it is one that can be practiced at home.

How to administer. You will need an oil bubbler along with a tube that runs from the exhaust to the patient. It's most common to use an adapted oxygen mask for ozone inhalation. Fill the oil bubbler so that the oil is three to four inches above the end of the straw where the ozone enters the bubbler. Connect the ozone generator to the center stem of the oil bubbler so that the ozone runs down into the oil and bubbles up through it. Next, connect the oxygen mask or other applicator that will be held near the patient's mouth to the offset (exhaust) port on the bubbler. If your generator allows, run it at a flow rate of ½ - ¾ LPM and a concentration of 40–50 µg/ml for 5 to 8 minutes. This high flow rate and concentration will allow you to quickly provide a good dose of ozonides. If your generator doesn't allow for you to produce a high concentration at a high flow rate, then set it at ¼ LPM and allow for a longer treatment of up to 20 minutes if possible. Most nonadjustable ozone generators will produce between 20–40 µg/ml at this setting.

Tips for nebulizing:

- Replace the oil when it becomes thick. Failure to do so could result in breathing in ozone. You should NEVER smell ozone while you are doing this treatment.
- Before using oil for the first time, bubble ozone through the oil for an hour. This will help to saturate the oil so that ozonides and peroxides are ready to be released during your first treatment.
- Although other oils can be used, organic virgin olive oil is the oil of choice for this method. Oils with fewer double bonds are not a good option as they may not convert the ozone to ozonides.

SUMMARY

There is a lot of information in this chapter, which you can revisit as a resource as needed. I don't know that there are any clinics that utilize every single method of ozone administration, but it's important to be able to administer ozone in a variety of ways as the situation demands, and a clinician must be able to utilize both systemic and local administration methods. Each of these categories includes one or more ways to administer ozone:

- Oils
- Fluids
- Insufflations
- Injections
- In the blood
- Inhalation

Choosing the right administration method and then properly administering ozone is key to a successful treatment, so make sure you understand what you are doing before you begin. If you don't feel confident to begin, attending a veterinary ozone training course like the one offered by O3Vets is a great way to build that confidence.

Chapter 5

Conditions and How to Treat Them

During the past decade, contrary to all expectations, it has been demonstrated that the judicious application of ozone in chronic infectious diseases, vasculopathies, orthopedics and even dentistry has yielded such striking results that it is deplorable that the medical establishment continues to ignore ozone therapy.

DR. VELIO BOCCI

"My name is Pamela Ruby-Russel, and this is Dudley Russel-Linter." Before me sat a woman pushing 60 with a red beret which told me she was an artist. The boy that sat on her lap wore a red sweater . . . and that was all he wore, only, he wasn't a boy. He was a fluffy, white pup who Mrs. Ruby-Russel rescued from Mexico. From his collar dangled a number of aluminum tags with enough information to satisfy the CIA. He sat with a slight grin on his face, letting me know that, even in this setting with the veterinarian ready to pounce, he had it good.

"Dudley was diagnosed with T-cell, high grade Lymphoma back in April of 2013, and he has been receiving O3UV treatments since the day after his diagnosis," said Pamela. Dudley was ten years old when diagnosed with lymphoma.

Initially things looked bleak as he was given three to six weeks to live. After his diagnosis, Pamela immediately took him to Dr. Margo Roman who started him on a journey to support his immune system. A huge part of that journey was the addition of ozone and ultraviolet blood irradiation to his treatment schedule. To the amazement of other veterinarians who were not familiar with these therapeutic modalities, Dudley went into remission and lived for two and a half healthy years, which is one of the longest periods of remission for a dog with T-cell Lymphoma. During this time, he received monthly maintenance treatments, which contributed to a superior quality of life for Dudley.

Into my inbox come a steady stream of emails asking whether ozone would be helpful in curing a particular illness. The emails come from pet owners and veterinarians alike, locating across the globe, ranging from South Africa to France to the Philippines. Most of my answers look similar, although some of the data changes. I usually say "yes" but with a caveat because many are looking for a miracle. Ozone is not a miracle in a syringe just waiting to be released into the tissue and cure animals of all their ailments. If that's what you're looking for, then keep looking.

If you're looking for a piece of the health puzzle that could have a significant impact, then you've found it in ozone therapy. It may be *the* piece you've been missing, and, for many, that's exactly what it is.

Now, let's look closely at the various conditions that have benefited from ozone therapy.

PREVENTATIVE USE

Just as an athlete can't wait until the day of the race to train, we can't wait until our animals are sick and then work on their health. Administering ozone therapy as a way to prevent illness needs to be a way of life. As we have already seen, it works to precondition our cells so they're ready and able to resist disease when it comes. What a great benefit.

One way to increase the value of ozone therapy in the clinic is to offer preventative treatments as part of the pet's wellness checkup. These can be scheduled every six months for healthy patients to keep a pet in optimum health and head off any disease before it starts. For pets who have had a chronic illness such as cancer, monthly treatments would be better. Because we are not treating any particular disease when we treat preventatively, use a systemic method of administration such as rectal insufflation, Major Autohemotherapy, or subcutaneous saline.

INJURY

One of the first times I saw ozone used was to treat a bite wound. The veterinarian ozonated water, drew it into a syringe, and lavaged the wound. External wounds such as abrasions, lacerations, contusions, bite wounds, and degloving wounds are most successfully treated by limb bagging, lavaging them with an ozonated fluid, or using a topical ozone product such as Pet Liniment 10%. Often, a combination of these administration options will be used. In many cases the veterinarian will lavage the wound with fluid and then send the client home with the topical product to apply twice a day for the next few weeks. There is a two-fold benefit to this approach as ozone is both able to disinfect the wound and stimulate healing.

Injuries that are generally internal—including a ruptured cruciate and torn meniscus, spinal compression, broken bones, and sprains—are most successfully treated with Prolo+Ozone injections. I talk more about this treatment in chapter six where we deal with combo treatments like Prolo+Ozone.

SURGERY

Ozonated saline will be worth its weight in gold to the surgeon. Powerful anti-infection properties make it a perfect solution for lavaging organs, tissue, and incisions during and after surgery. Besides the ozone generator, the fluid bubbler will provide more value to the veterinarian than any other ozone accessory. Remember, the anti-infection properties are just a part of the reason that ozone is important here. Ozone will also help bring nutrients to the area and produce growth factors that speed the healing process. Keeping a flask of saline handy and recharging it with ozone at the appropriate time will make this process efficient.

In the case of broken bones, or deep lacerations that require surgery or stitches, injecting Prolo+Ozone into an area during surgery may speed the healing process even more. Of course, using ozone during surgery will be a more expensive treatment for the client, so this option should be approved beforehand.

DENTISTRY

"In my view, it's almost malpractice not to use ozone in dentistry." Dr. John Augspurger is a biological dentist in the Denver area with a bent toward ozone therapy. The statement he made to me that day shows just how vital he considers ozone to be for his practice. Gum disease, sores, cavities, infections, oral surgeries, and other oral conditions can benefit tremendously from ozone therapy. In this case also, ozonated fluids are the most common way to apply ozone, but gas injections into the area of concern can be even more effective. Ozonated fluid can be used before, during, and after cleanings and extractions with an emphasis on reducing or eliminating antibiotics which only disrupt the healthy microflora of the mouth. A third application is to use a product such as Hydrogel 15% which uses ozonated sunflower seed oil as the active ingredient and is formulated specifically for oral use. One of the benefits of Hydrogel 15% is that it can be sent home with the client and applied twice a day in the comfort of their home.

AUTOIMMUNE

A dysfunctional immune system is the cause of a host of diseases, including polyarthritis, allergies, and skin problems. Bluebell Chamberlin's case stands out to me. Bluebell was a sixteen-month-old Blue Merle Sheltie at the time of her treatment. Among other things, she had previously been treated with a number of drugs, including Dexamethasone IV, Baytril IM, and oral Prednisone. The treatments never had a lasting effect and her condition worsened. Eventually, her owners brought her to a veterinarian who utilized ozone therapy as well as another novel integrative therapy called Ultraviolet Blood Irradiation. Bluebell was treated using Major Autohemotherapy plus Ultraviolet (O3UV), and after just four treatments, her condition began to improve. Within a few months of beginning treatment, Bluebell had a full recovery and was able to live without medications or pain. Granted, the treatment that saved Bluebell was a combination of both ozone therapy and Ultraviolet Blood Irradiation, which we'll talk about later, but the powerful, combined effect of these two modalities was unquestionable.

Most of the time a systemic administration method such as MAHT (Major Autohemotherapy), subcutaneous saline, or rectal insufflation will be used to treat autoimmune conditions, but I want to emphasize that there is an added benefit to combining MAHT with mAHT (minor Autohemotherapy) as well. If you really want to go all out, a great treatment for autoimmune conditions is O3UV immediately followed by mAHT. It really doesn't take much effort to administer mAHT when doing MAHT. Just take the last little amount of blood—usually 1-3 ml—shake it vigorously for 20 seconds and inject it into the muscle instead of putting it back into the vein.

INFECTION

Infections can occur in any part of the body. Ozone can be applied to any part of the body, and because of its powerful anti-infection properties, it can be a champion treatment for an animal struggling with a local or systemic infection. Viral, bacterial, or fungal infections often require harsh antibiotics that produce nasty side effects. By direct oxidation of the pathogen, increased oxygenation, and immune system activation, ozone can often effectively eliminate the infection. Ear infections are common and can be extremely stubborn. Infectious skin diseases can cause a ghastly appearance and poor quality of life for the pet and the owner. Urinary tract infections can be painful and hard to care for. Other common infections such as parvovirus, Lyme disease, and kennel cough should all include ozone as a part of the treatment plan. I won't mention every infection here because it would take too much paper but understand that ozone therapy is a great treatment for infections. It works.

CANCER

About 25% of dogs and 20% of cats get cancer. It's likely that you have had or will have a pet with this dreaded disease. If you're a veterinarian, a large percentage of your practice is probably dedicated to diagnosing and treating cancer. Even with all of our medical and technological advances in the last century, cancer is still winning the battle.

In a lecture by Dr. Betsy Hershey, she discussed the following case:

> Izzy was diagnosed at age three with osteosarcoma. The owner didn't want to amputate or do any conventional therapies, so we elected to try ozone therapy. Izzy had complete regression of the tumor after about six months of therapy. We continued with maintenance treatments every two to three months, and she remained in remission for four years after diagnosis. To get that amount of time without amputation and chemotherapy is pretty remarkable because you usually get about a year to two years with those traditional treatments.

While ozone therapy is not *the* answer for cancer, it is one of the keys to successfully battling this disease. Dr. Silvia Menendez has this to say, "Although ozone therapy is not able to eradicate the tumor completely, it improves the quality of life, reduces metastasis, increases the survival of animals, and even reduces the adverse effects of chemo and radiotherapy."[36]

If you skipped through chapter three of this book, go back and carefully read about how ozone works. Understanding the mechanisms of ozone therapy will keep you using it even when you aren't seeing the effects as quickly as you would like. Here's my point: ozone therapy may not cure cancer like it did for Izzy, but it will usually slow the disease and provide a better quality of life for the animal.

Dr. Judith Shoemaker made the following statement about the use of ozone therapy in her practice during an interview I had with her:

> It reduces the amount of chemotherapy that I've had to use in my practice by at least 25%. I have animals that cannot tolerate carboplatin in therapeutic doses, but carboplatin works like a champ concurrently with ozone. I can use one quarter the dose and get the same effect or more without side effects when I do ozone as well. I work with a lot of oncologists who tell me, "I don't know what you're doing but keep doing it because this animal is getting better." Even animals who have become resistant to the effectiveness of chemotherapy, when you add ozone in, it often becomes effective again.

We would do well to listen to the advice of Dr. Shoemaker and not hesitate to apply ozone therapy to all types of cancer cases. Besides the anecdotal information, research has been conducted on various types of cancers, including carcinomas, tumors, leukemia, and sarcomas. The weight of evidence tips the balance decisively in the favor of ozone therapy as an important treatment.

In general, there's no better way to treat cancer with ozone therapy than to employ O3UV. The powerful combination of ozone and ultraviolet light can provide the knockout punch necessary to put the terrible disease behind you. If you're doing this treatment at home, rectal insufflation is the way to go. Local tumors should also be treated with a local application of ozone, such as subcutaneous saline, ozone oil, ozone gas injections, or mAHT injected around or into the tumor.

Until more evidence is provided to the contrary, the decision as to which method to use isn't as important as just applying ozone.

CONTRAINDICATIONS

At a lunch in 2017, Dr. Judith Shoemaker said, "I have never in twenty-five years had an inappropriate reaction to ozone." Using the word "contraindication" means that we are not able to treat a disease because the negative effects would outweigh the positive effects. I'm not aware of a disease for which that holds true with ozone therapy. However, bleeding disorders are a category of disease where we need to take precautions.

With the following conditions, the blood doesn't clot properly, and bleeding occurs very easily:

- Hemophilia
- Thrombocytopenia
- Hemorrhagic conditions

Because ozone therapy improves the blood flow properties, these conditions can worsen when applying ozone.

When I've discussed this with my veterinary friends and ozone trainers, their response has been that they don't avoid using ozone with these conditions, but that they start with a lower dose. It may be wise to use a method that doesn't require drawing blood, and it goes without saying that if you do draw blood, don't use an anticoagulant.

If I haven't mentioned the specific disease that you are interested in treating with ozone, don't despair. My friend Dr. Albert Nunez had this to say:

> In our cancer patients, the difference is day and night, but it's not just for cancer. It's for so many things. We'll bubble up saline and put it in bladders, we'll put it in sinuses. For all of our surgical fluids, we have a bubbler of ozonated fluids that flushes all our lavages, wounds, all our orthopedics, and anything infected. With ozone you'll see the tissue change right in front of you which is really instant gratification.

I understand the skepticism out there because spending millions of dollars to formulate a drug specifically for one disease has become a way of life in our American healthcare system. That doesn't mean that the way we currently do things is the right way. In fact, I would argue, along with many others, that our healthcare system and the way we treat disease is broken. The bad news is that because people will always oversee healthcare, it will always have problems. The good news is that you can help lead the way toward a more holistic, less complicated, and more effective way of doing medicine that gets to root causes instead of masking symptoms.

SUMMARY

Because of its ability to reduce inflammation and promote cellular oxygenation, ozone therapy is a powerful veterinary tool that can help almost every patient. In most cases, ozone therapy is a non-specific treatment that helps the body heal itself. This is why it can be successfully implemented as a primary or adjunct treatment for so many disease processes. If you take a look at the ISCO3 library of ozone therapy research at Zotero.org, you'll see the general focus of the research as it pertains to various diseases and areas within medicine. Here are some of the results:

- Musculoskeletal – 568 results
- Dental and Oral – 298 results
- Neurological – 127 results
- Cardiovascular – 127 results
- Infections – 126 results
- Oncology – 113 results
- Gynecology/Obstetrics – 80 results
- Endocrinology – 70 results
- Immunology/Allergies – 68 results
- Dermatology – 63 results

As you can see, there is no shortage of studies when it comes to the multidisciplinary use of ozone. Often, the limiting factor is the experience and vision of the veterinarian and not the safety or effectiveness of ozone therapy.

Chapter 6

The Multimodal Approach: Combining Ozone with Other Treatments

Ozone really helps the effectiveness of all of my other therapies.

DR. JUDITH SHOEMAKER

In a scientific article available on PubMed entitled "Multimodal Therapy: Overview of Principles, Barriers and Opportunities," we find this statement:

> For example, in PD and Alzheimer's disease (AD), protein misfolding and dysfunction in how proteins are trafficked and cleared, neuroinflammation, mitochondrial dysfunction, oxidative stress, and other aging pathways have all been implicated and may need to be targeted in combination.

As a side note, it's incredible that ozone therapy deals directly with many of the problems identified in this short statement. Might it be that ozone therapy could be a central piece of the puzzle in the treatment of Alzheimer's and Parkinson's? Preliminary research suggests that it may be.

Deep down, we know that treating disease isn't as easy as popping a pill. Even if that may help alleviate symptoms, there isn't a person alive who doesn't realize the benefits of clean water, nutritious food, frequent exercise, sufficient sleep, a good thought life, healthy relationships, etc. These things are medicine . . . the best kind of medicine.

Veterinarians who have taken a more holistic approach to treating patients are ahead of the curve. All veterinarians know these things are true, but most have not been trained to think and act in a way that would include these issues in the diagnosis and treatment plan. They may even mention some of these things as side issues that clients need to be aware of, but they haven't centered their treatment plans around them. What would happen if our entire country was made up of veterinarians who adopted a multimodal, holistic mentality? Veterinary care would be transformed, and our pets would live longer, healthier lives. I guarantee it. But it's really the desire for a quick, inexpensive fix that drives the inability to solve the root cause of the disease. Positive change starts with me. It starts with you. It starts with us.

Part of the change we all long for is adopting a multimodal treatment plan that takes synergistic treatments and combines them to create a more powerful healing effect. The purpose of this chapter is to explore what we know about certain treatment combinations that include ozone therapy. Although there are more, the ones I have chosen to discuss are ultraviolet blood irradiation (UBI) and injection therapies, including PRP, prolo, and stem cells. I'll also briefly discuss a couple of other treatments including acupuncture and chemo/radiation.

We'll explore some of the ways that ozone therapy and each of the above modalities are used in combination and what you can expect. This will be a quick introduction and not a thorough exposition. When I talk about the needed supplies and equipment for each treatment, I will not be mentioning the ozone side of the equation as we have already covered that. Keep in mind that the guidelines on how to do the treatments in this book are not official protocols and should not take the place of the manufacturer's instructions or your own veterinary judgment.

ULTRAVIOLET BLOOD IRRADIATION

UBI is my favorite treatment to combine with ozone therapy. We'll spend a little more time here than on the other modalities. That may be because I got my introduction to ozone therapy while working to develop UBI equipment and protocols, but it's also because there is a great deal of scientific evidence demonstrating that ozone and UBI are more powerful when performed in combination than when performed separately.

Sunlight can heal. Part of the light we receive from the sun is ultraviolet. In the 1800s, the healing power of these special ultraviolet rays was discovered. In 1904, the Danish physician Niels Finsen used ultraviolet light to treat skin conditions and was eventually awarded the Nobel Prize. UBI was developed by scientist Emmett Knott in the 1920s and was subsequently used through the 1950s to treat many diseases, including septicemia, pneumonia, tuberculosis, arthritis, and even asthma, but the first studies were actually carried out on dogs moribund with infection. All the dogs treated with UBI recovered while many in the control group died. This led to numerous studies carried out by a few doctors. However, with the discovery of antibiotics, UBI almost disappeared from use in the United States. After its disappearance here, UBI was more heavily utilized in Russia and other Eastern countries where many of the studies were performed.

I remember speaking to an elderly medical doctor who told me about her father's experience in a Florida hospital back in the 1940s. He had begun using UBI as a treatment just prior to the widespread use of antibiotics. As the excitement over these "miracle drugs" bubbled, this doctor was ordered by the hospital administration to "get that machine out of here." It had been concluded that our need for technology such as UBI had run its course. Now, with the ever-increasing issue of antibiotic-resistant pathogens and the ever-present side effects of medications, it has become apparent that other options are necessary.

What it is. UBI is an immune modulating treatment that uses ultraviolet light to treat blood. To administer a treatment, a small amount of blood is withdrawn from the patient and then mixed with saline to dilute. That mixture is then channeled through a quartz tube and past ultraviolet light where it absorbs the photons from that light. Once treated, it is reintroduced back into the bloodstream.

In 2015, I visited the Wellman Center for Photomedicine at Massachusetts General Hospital, the largest research facility in the world dedicated to studying the use of light as medicine. At the time, Michael Hamblin, Ph.D., was the principal investigator there, and he was also an associate professor at the Harvard Medical School. The work he has done on the use of light in medicine is astounding and, if it were not for his humble demeanor, he would have made me feel grossly inadequate.

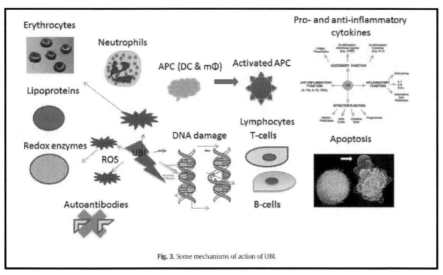

Fig. 3. Some mechanisms of action of UBI

Wu X, Hu X, Hamblin MR. Ultraviolet blood irradiation: Is it time to remember "the cure that time forgot"? J Photochem Photobiol B. 2016 Apr;157:89-96. doi: 10.1016/j.jphotobiol.2016.02.007. Epub 2016 Feb 5. PMID: 26894849; PMCID: PMC4783265.

In 2016, I had the privilege of working with Dr. Hamblin to develop a clinical evaluation report on UBI. Working on that report and learning directly from Dr. Hamblin brought me a deeper appreciation of how UBI works, but it's complicated. Anything dealing with the immune system is complicated, and anyone who tries to convince you of the contrary is either lying or ignorant. The more we uncover how a treatment works, the more we realize that each treatment has a multiplicity of effects we weren't aware of at the outset. Although much has been discovered about how UBI works, much is yet to be understood.

What do we know at this point? We know that UBI works upon the principle of hormesis. The basic concept of hormesis is that a small dose of a stressor can stimulate a favorable biological response. So ultraviolet light, just like ozone, can be beneficial in the right amounts because it places stress on the body that activates certain immune cells or inhibits their activation based on the body's needs and the condition being treated. Here are some key takeaways regarding UBI.

- It works like an auto-vaccine to trigger the production of antibodies that destroy pathogens.
- It can have an immunosuppressive effect by reducing lymphocyte reaction.
- It enhances phagocytic activity, thus reducing dead and toxic cells from the patient.
- It can reduce free radical damage and elevate the activity of antioxidant enzymes.

It makes sense to mention extracorporeal photopheresis (ECP) here. ECP is an immunotherapy developed in the 1980s to treat cutaneous T-cell lymphoma by Yale dermatologist Dr. Richard Edelson. The process involves spinning out the blood and isolating white blood cells, treating them with a photosensitizing agent called Psoralen, and then exposing them to UVA light before returning them to the body. This photopheresis process produces an immunomodulatory effect by stimulating a stronger immune response when necessary or downregulating that same immune system in the case of autoimmune conditions.

Why you should combine it with ozone. In 2014, I attended an ozone therapy conference put on by the Mexican Association of Ozone Therapy.[37] Dr. Frank Shallenberger was a speaker at that conference and is one of the most respected ozone doctors in the United States. It was at that conference when we asked him why he combined ozone with UBI that he told us this story:

> A number of years back, I received a patient at my door who had basically been sent home to die. She was full of infections, had tachycardia, 33 breaths per minute, a 103° fever and her O_2 saturation was 86. I too thought she was going to die. I tried treating her with ozone with no

success. I purchased a biophotonic (UBI) device and gave her one 60 cc treatment. She had a total turn around within 24 hours. Everything got better. It was not perfect, and so I gave her a second treatment. It was absolutely remarkable! The biophotonic therapy (Ultraviolet Blood Irradiation) cured her in just three days. Biophotonic therapy does something different . . . it definitely does something very good and very different than ozone. I have done this for years and would never go back to just using ozone in blood as a therapy.

There is anecdotal evidence that it works, but we have more than mere anecdotes as well. In the 1990s, a Canadian biotech company, Vasogen, patented a device called the Celacade and developed a treatment known as Immune Modulation Therapy (IMT). To perform a treatment, about 10-20 ml of blood was drawn from the patient and introduced into the device where it was treated with UVC light, ozone, and sometimes heat before being injected intramuscularly. The method used by Vasogen closely mimics mAHT. The goal of this treatment was to produce oxidative stress that would trigger an anti-inflammatory immunomodulation response. Unfortunately, a huge phase III randomized, double-blind, placebo study failed to produce the desired results, which caused Vasogen stock to plummet. But they left behind a treasure trove of studies that show that the combination of ozone and ultraviolet are synergistic and produce a more powerful response by:

- Inhibiting the aggregation of blood platelets (#5591457)
- Increasing nitric oxide (#5834030)
- Preconditioning the body against stress (#6136308)
- Reducing atherosclerosis and inhibiting progression of atherosclerotic lesions (#6669965)

- Inhibiting inflammatory cytokine secretion (#7122208)

You can go look up these patent studies at www.uspto.gov. You can also go to www.pubmed.gov and search "Vasogen" to read about their IMT.

The inventors of this technology understood the benefit of subjecting the patient's blood to stressors (heat, ozone, and UV light) that produced an auto-vaccine which could trigger one or more of the above responses. The research was extensive throughout the '90s and into the 21st century as Vasogen proved that controlled amounts of stress could redefine the body's terrain and produce a healing effect.

Although they were looking for a condition that would be a slam dunk for their IMT, we look at the data in an altogether different light today. We recognize that there isn't a silver bullet cure, but that this treatment is a crucial piece of the puzzle when it comes to correcting underlying health conditions. But correcting these issues is only part of the problem. We must also be willing to implement lifestyle changes related to diet, exercise, detoxification, emotional well-being, etc. that will produce lasting results. O3UV can be a major healing catalyst, but you must be the agent for change.

What you need. The central piece is the UBI machine. It consists of an irradiation chamber surrounded by ultraviolet lamps that irradiate the blood sample as it passes through. This chamber should be designed with reflective materials because it can get up to 20% more energy into the blood.

The Chimp UV is designed by O3Vets and utilizes UVA, UVB, and UVC lamps to treat the blood. Each of these wavelengths produces a slightly different effect, with UVA being the least germicidal and UVC the most. We've already heard about extracorporeal photopheresis, which uses

UVA, and of IMT, which uses UVC. UVB is a wavelength most commonly used to treat skin conditions such as Psoriasis. The combination of all three wavelengths in treatment ensures that the patient benefits from the unique properties of each wavelength.

The UBI device is always accompanied by something called a cuvette. The cuvette that's paired with the Chimp UV is a round quartz tube with a spiral insert that helps mix the blood as it goes through the irradiation chamber. The quartz material is a special type that allows the ultraviolet light to pass through and absorb into the blood. Other types of glass and plastic materials have a poor transmission ratio that blocks most of the UV energy and would lead to an ineffective treatment. Flexible IV lines are attached to each side of the quartz tube and terminate in a luer-lock connection. This allows the user to attach the cuvette to other accessories that may be necessary to perform a treatment or to attach the cuvette to itself to form a closed-loop system. The cuvette comes in a sterile package and is intended for single use. I never recommend cleaning out something that has had blood products in it because it is impossible to verify the sterility of the product once cleaned, and it could produce an infection in the patient if it isn't perfectly sterile. A 250 ml blood bag is also provided by O3Vets and is necessary when treating any animal over 20 pounds. It is a sterile, single-use bag designed to hold the blood and saline that will be treated with ozone and ultraviolet light. It connects directly to the cuvette to form a closed-loop system and has a needle port that can be used to inject the fluid into the bag. Video protocols on how to perform the treatment are available through O3Vets.

Apart from the normal supplies already in a veterinary clinic, the final piece of equipment needed is an infusion pump. I find that most veterinarians already have one of these. Most of the time your pump will work well with the O3Vets cuvette lines.

How to administer. A more detailed protocol is available through O3Vets, but we'll walk through the basics of how to treat an animal over 20 pounds with O3UV. For animals under 20 pounds, the protocol is similar but does not include the use of the blood bag.

Infuse saline into the blood bag at a rate of four parts saline to one part blood (4:1). Heparinize a syringe with 50 units per milliliter of blood and draw 2-4 ml of blood per 10 pounds of patient body weight. If the animal has a bleeding disorder, do not use an anticoagulant. Infuse the blood into the blood bag with the saline. Pull up 40µg/ml of ozone at two parts ozone to one part blood (2:1) and infuse that into the bag. Gently rock the bag to mix the contents, and then hang it on an IV pole. Connect the cuvette to the bag and allow it to fill with the mixture. Place the cuvette into the lid of the Chimp UV and turn it on. Place the cuvette line into the infusion pump. After setting the correct volume, run it at 360 ml/hr. Draw all the solution out of the bag and reinfuse it intravenously back to the patient.

Intra-Articular Injections

Ozone injections have been used to treat herniated discs, spinal damage, degenerative joints, arthritis, sports injuries, and more, but combining ozone with these injections is a more powerful way to treat them. Intra-articular injections in this context refer to injections that stimulate healing and/or reduce inflammation. Some of these injectable therapies will fall under the category of orthobiologics—the use of a biological material to treat musculoskeletal issues, but all these therapies should be considered regenerative medicine.

Before I started researching this area, my intent was to discuss the two elements I was familiar with, dextrose and platelet-rich plasma (PRP). As I researched, I discovered that these were not the only injectable elements that had been studied alongside ozone therapy. There was at least one study that utilized stem cells and ozone together. Hyaluronic acid (HA) is also a very common element that's been used over dextrose and PRP to treat similar conditions with good success. I was also amazed to see that there had been studies that used HA along with ozone therapy. Based on my research, it's too early to say whether PRP, HA, dextrose, stem cells, Prolozone®, or a combination of these would be most effective.

As we move through this section, I'll do my best to lay out the data and make sense of it. Let's move through these injection treatments one by one.

Prolotherapy. If we use the term "prolotherapy" loosely to indicate the use of a stimulant to induce the inflammatory healing cascade, we would have to say that prolotherapy has its origins in ancient history. However, the first use of prolotherapy similar to what we use today was in the 1830s by Alfred Velpeau, MD. A more sophisticated approach was developed by Dr. Earl Gedney in the 1930s. Today, prolotherapy is understood as an injection therapy that stimulates a healing response and is most commonly used to treat musculoskeletal disorders. Both Velpeau and Gedney used dextrose as the injectable solution, but there are several elements that can be used.

What it is. According to Prolotherapycollege.org, another definition of prolotherapy is as follows:

> Prolotherapy is a recognized orthopedic procedure that stimulates the body's healing processes to strengthen and repair injured and painful joints and connective tissue. It

95

is based on the fact that when ligaments or tendons are stretched or torn, the joint they are holding destabilizes and can become painful. Prolotherapy, with its unique ability to directly address the cause of the instability, can repair the weakened sites and produce new collagen tissue, resulting in permanent stabilization of the joint.[38]

Most of the scientific information available on prolotherapy utilizes dextrose as the primary injectable solution, but it often combines that with lidocaine. There's current debate and uncertainty regarding what solution and concentrations are best. For example, some prolotherapists believe that the more likely myotoxic effects of lidocaine make it a less desirable product as compared to procaine.[39]

Another debated question is the concentration of dextrose and lidocaine, which was explored in a study out of the *Korean Journal of Pain* where the authors advocate for 1% dextrose and 0.1% lidocaine as opposed to the normal doses of 10-25% dextrose and 1% lidocaine.[40]

Although these questions are still unanswered, and more work needs to be done to discover the best option, we have good data indicating that a variety of solutions and concentrations are effective and safe. This systematic review and meta-analysis[41] was published in 2021 and provides a good synopsis on the available literature. In short, they found that dextrose prolotherapy is comparable to the effect of PRP or steroid injections.

A variation of prolotherapy used by many human and veterinary practitioners but that has little evidence to support its use has been developed by Dr. Frank Shallenberger. In fact, he coined the term Prolozone® and registered a trademark on it. But Dr. Shallenberger's brand of injection therapy goes beyond the combination of ozone and prolo. In a 2011 paper, Dr. Shallenberger wrote the following:

Prolozone is a technique that combines the principles of neural therapy, Prolotherapy and ozone therapy. It involves injecting combinations of procaine, anti-inflammatory medications, homeopathics, vitamins, minerals, proliferates and ozone/oxygen gas into degenerated or injured joints and into areas of pain. The result of this combination is nothing short of remarkable in that damaged tissues can be regenerated, and otherwise untreatable pain can be permanently cured.[42]

When I started my journey into ozone therapy, Prolozone® was the first injection therapy that I was introduced to and, consequently, we've taught this technique at our O3Vets training courses. Although it is possible that this is the most effective technique, we don't know for certain because comparative studies have not been done that utilize all the elements suggested by Dr. Shallenberger.

There are two versions of the solution that Dr. Shallenberger recommends depending on the condition being treated and the severity of the disease. For conditions that exhibit excessive inflammation, he recommends what he has labeled as his "anti-inflammatory solution." Once a few treatments have been effectively administered using this solution and the inflammation has decreased, he recommends the use of his "proliferative solution," which includes morrhuate sodium. The morrhuate sodium irritates the area and produces a temporary and controlled inflammatory response. This short-term response is localized in the injection area, initiating the release of cytokines, which bring other immune cells, hormones, and nutrients to heal the damaged area. The use of ozone restores oxygen to areas that are naturally deprived because of trauma. The increase of oxygen and oxygen utilization in an area of pain or injury is a necessary and crucial step in the healing process. All degenerative diseases can be traced back to a lack of oxygen at the cellular level, and there is no better way to oxygenate than to use ozone.

Veterinarians are notorious for translating protocols from human medicine and using their clinical judgment to determine how to treat a patient. This may be a case where that is warranted, but I will leave the final decision to you.

Why it should be combined. Whether you choose to use traditional prolotherapy with ozone, Dr. Shallenberger's Prolozone® injection, or your own concoction, you must be confident that the various components are not counteracting each other and that you are providing the best possible outcome for your patient. Prolotherapy works by stimulating the body to lay down new tissue in the weakened area by producing a mild inflammatory response. This inflammatory response encourages growth of new ligaments or tendon fibers that strengthen the structure. When ozone is added to this injection, it increases the healing potential in a few specific ways. First, it increases oxygen utilization, which helps break the cycle of chronic pain and degeneration so that the cells and tissue can heal.[43] Second, it stimulates the production of growth factors, which are signaling proteins that stimulate cell growth and tissue repair. Third, ozone works as an analgesic to reduce pain, which traditional prolotherapy doesn't do.

In a study published in 2015, a clinical trial[44] compared the results of hypertonic dextrose versus ozone injections to treat knee osteoarthritis (KOA). Patients were separated into two groups with one group receiving ozone injections and the other receiving prolo injections. The results indicated that both treatments "can be effectively used in the nonoperative management of patients with KOA." But there was no statistical significance between the two groups. Unfortunately, the study did not include the combination of ozone and prolo together nor did it use anything but dextrose for the prolo solution. It's disappointing that there still isn't much scientific information available on the combination of prolotherapy and ozone therapy beyond what Dr. Shallenberger has provided from his own experience. There are currently thousands of doctors and veterinarians around the world who are using this technique, but most of the scientific data available is on either the injection of ozone into a joint *or* the injection of prolo solution, but not both.

When discussing what we should be treating, Dr. Shallenberger states, "The primary criterion for selecting a patient for Prolozone® is pain. If it hurts, Prolozone® should be tried." In the veterinary field, I've found that it's most common to treat soft tissue injuries of which cruciate tears are at the top of the list. Beyond these, osteoarthritis (OA) or just general pain are also great candidates.

What you need.

- Ozone therapy equipment
- Prolo solution (dextrose, lidocaine, etc.)
- Hypodermic needle
- 3-10 ml syringe

The beauty of prolotherapy is that it's inexpensive to start. There is no equipment that you need to purchase, and the solution itself can be less than a dollar (if you go with just dextrose) to $10 per injection (if you purchase a premade solution from a company like Drug Crafters[45]). Either way, your investment is minimal. Besides your solution, you'll need a needle and a couple of syringes. The syringe and needle size will depend on the joint you're injecting and the size of the animal, but the most common size used is a 10 ml syringe and a 27 g x 1½" needle.

How to administer. All of these regenerative injections should be performed by an experienced veterinarian. You must be a veterinarian with training in both anatomy and injection technique. Before you give the injection, you'll need to shave and prep the area. Most veterinarians will sedate the patient, while some will do the injection using the prolo solution with lidocaine or procaine as a local numbing agent.

AMOUNT	INGREDIENT
1cc	B12
5cc	0.9% Saline
1.2cc	50% Dextrose
4cc	2% Procaine

The most common joints to inject are the knees, so it's normal to become quite comfortable with those injections while not reaching that same comfort level with the rest of the joints.

Once the patient and the area are prepped and ready, you'll need to draw up your prolo solution into a syringe. If you're mixing your own solution, utilize the proper concentrations and sanitary techniques to ensure a safe and effective treatment. In a separate syringe, draw up the ozone. First, administer an intra-articular injection of the solution. Leave the needle in the joint. Using a hemostat, hold the needle and gently twist the prolo syringe off and then attach the ozone syringe. You can now inject the ozone through the same needle that was used for the prolo solution. Some veterinarians will also do a few periarticular injections, which may help strengthen the ligaments and tissue around the joint.

In the systematic review cited earlier, it was most common to do three injections each spaced a month apart. Another meta-analysis on prolotherapy for OA stated, "Pooling data from two RCTs, we report that peri- and intra-articular hypertonic dextrose knee injections in three to five sessions have statistically significant and clinically relevant effect."[46] The effects seem to reduce pain for up to a year, but it may be possible to see long-term benefits as well. I've discussed the issue of how many injections should be done with veterinarians, and it seems most common to do one to three injections spaced from two weeks to one month apart. Outcomes will vary depending on the condition being treated, but 60–80% is an expected efficacy rate.[47]

Platelet-rich plasma (PRP). PRP injections have really taken off since 2008 and are being used in a variety of conditions. For our purposes here, we're going to focus on the use of PRP for musculoskeletal injuries. Groups like the Veterinary Orthopedic Sports Medicine Group in Maryland[48] focus very heavily on this particular injection. If I'm honest, this is probably the most popular of the injections that we'll discuss in this book.

Last year there were over one thousand PRP studies published on PubMed alone. Of course, with OA being the most commonly diagnosed joint disease in animals, there are many studies that focus on this. Just to give an example, in 2021, a study entitled "Platelet-rich plasma therapy in dogs with bilateral hip osteoarthritis" demonstrated that intra-articular injections of police dogs helped to reduce pain and improve the dog's ability to function normally. When I talk with veterinarians about these types of injections, HA injections are minimally effective; prolotherapy injections are an unknown; and stem cells are too expensive. PRP, however, is right on the edge of being affordable and produces results similar to stem cells.

What it is. PRP falls into the category of regenerative medicine. Regenerative medicine harnesses the body's innate healing power in an effort to regenerate tissue or organs that have been damaged by disease or trauma. PRP uses the body's own cells to heal damage to the musculoskeletal system primarily through increasing growth factors.

In the 1960s and '70s, experimental usage of PRP was taking place in the United States.[49],[50] In the 1980s, dental specialists used PRP during surgery to reduce blood loss and speed bone healing.[51] It wasn't until the twenty-first century that studies investigated PRP injections for injured joints and backs. In fact, the term "orthobiologics" describes injections like PRP and stem cells ("ortho" refers to bone and "biologics" refers to naturally derived substances from the body).

PRP has become more than just a treatment for musculoskeletal injuries. Its usage now includes cardiac surgery, pediatric surgery, gynecology, urology, plastic surgery, ophthalmology,[52] and dermatology.[53] Study in these areas didn't take off until after 2008, but advancements in understanding since that time have led to more successful treatments.

In veterinary medicine, PRP is generally used to treat horses and dogs, but it can be used on any animal from which enough blood can be drawn. Although using PRP for cats isn't common, an interesting study[54] was performed to determine the effectiveness of centrifuging feline blood. The volume of blood taken from cats was about 13 ml. The results show it was difficult to get the desired concentration of platelets and that aggregation is a concern that needs to be addressed.

Why it should be combined. There is a growing interest in the use of ozone with PRP injections. During our last International Veterinary Ozone Therapy Summit in Florida, Dr. Jean Joaquim, President of Bioethicus in Brazil and head of the Brazilian Veterinary Ozone

Organization, talked about how they had discovered that mixing ozone with the platelets prior to injection activates the platelets and produces a more potent effect. The previous year, Dr. Calin Repciuc, from the Faculty of Veterinary Medicine at the University of Agricultural Sciences and Veterinary Medicine in Romania, joined us and delivered a lecture regarding wound healing. As I talked with him prior to that lecture, we hit on the topic of injecting ozone and PRP together. Here in the USA, it is more common to see these injections done separately, but Dr. Repciuc had particular interest in doing research to demonstrate that you should actually mix the two prior to injection.

A 2019 study[55] shows us that combining ozone with PRP injections has merit. The study states that "patients receiving ozone treatment are less likely to experience post-injection pain and are more likely to recover faster when compared to patients receiving PRP treatment alone." A study[56] published in 2021 compared ozonated PRP to PRP alone to expedite tendon-to-bone healing in rabbits. The results showed that both treatments were successful, but that the ozonated PRP treatment outperformed PRP alone.

What you need.

- Centrifuge
- PRP kit
- Syringes
- Needles
- General anesthesia setup

The initial setup for a centrifuge will run about $3,000–$6,000. The disposable PRP kit is where companies who sell this equipment make their money. The cost of those kits is between $150–$250, which has caused some resourceful veterinarians to look at using a blood draw tube and centrifuge. The benefit of using these tubes is that the cost decreases to less than one dollar for the tube, but the drawback is the decrease in platelet count.

A typical PRP system results in a 4- to 7-fold increase in platelets and a reduction of 85%–95% of the neutrophils and red blood cells. Using a blood tube to spin out the blood and draw out the thin layer of PRP while leaving the neutrophils and red blood cells behind can be very challenging. As you consider the cost/benefit ratio, you must ask yourself how many patients could benefit from these treatments if just one injection costs $400, the common charge at a veterinary office. In turn, the use of a blood tube will allow you to reduce the cost by at least $100.

While cost inevitably plays into the equation, the most important question regards efficacy. There is evidence indicating that the optimal increase of platelets is a 3- to 5-fold baseline. Additionally, the inclusion of neutrophils as well as red blood cells seems to be detrimental to the treatment outcome.[57] A consensus on whether blood tubes can be used has not been reached, but if you choose to go that route, you can find studies[58] that enumerate how it should be done. In the article "Principles and Methods of Preparation of Platelet-Rich Plasma: A Review and Author's Perspective," you'll find a wealth of helpful information that could increase your success regardless of the equipment that you use.

How to administer. The patient is usually put under general anesthesia prior to the blood draw. To perform a PRP injection, about 10-30 ml of the patient's blood is withdrawn (30 ml of blood will yield approximately 3-5 ml of PRP depending on whether some of the platelet poor plasma is drawn up as well). After the blood is drawn and mixed with an anticoagulant, it is put into a special container called a PRP kit and then placed in the centrifuge. The centrifuge is a mechanical device that spins at high speeds to separate the various components in the blood, making it possible to extract the desired component. A layer of PRP is drawn from the sample. A syringe of ozone gas is connected to the syringe of PRP using a female-to-female Luer-lock connector. The ozone is then infused into the PRP. Gently rock the syringe to ensure that all the ozone is absorbed, and then inject the ozonated PRP into the problem area.

Hyaluronic acid (HA). As I mentioned at the outset of this section on intra-articular injections, I didn't plan to discuss this treatment until I began seeing it come up repeatedly when looking at studies on PRP, ozone, and stem cells.

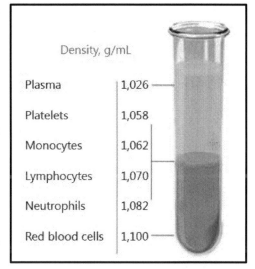

Density, g/mL	
Plasma	1,026
Platelets	1,058
Monocytes	1,062
Lymphocytes	1,070
Neutrophils	1,082
Red blood cells	1,100

Experimental studies on the use of HA started in the 1940s, but in OA. When this proved successful, human studies were initiated. In the late 1990s, HA became an FDA approved and commercially available product. Currently, HA stands alongside of corticosteroids as a common injection treatment for KOA.

What it is. HA is a product that our body produces that helps lubricate our joints. A synthetic version of this fluid has been developed and is used to treat KOA. Because HA injections supplement the naturally produced synovial fluid, this treatment is often referred to as Visco supplementation.[59] A classic effect of OA is the reduction in the viscoelastic properties of the synovial fluid, meaning the synovial fluid becomes runny and loses its elasticity. But more important than the supplementation of the synovial fluid is the effect that synthetic HA has to stimulate the production of endogenous HA.

A study[60] comparing PRP and hyaluronic acid demonstrated that both injections were statistically significant for up to two months. But only PRP had a significant ongoing effect beyond six months. Another study[61] showed similar results and helps support the conclusion that PRP has long-lasting effects beyond the effects of hyaluronic acid for treating KOA. One of the best ways to find out what treatment is better is to do a review of the current literature available. In 2020, a review[62] compared PRP and HA for treating KOA. It demonstrated that "mean improvement was significantly higher in the PRP group (44.7%) than the HA group (12.6%) for WOMAC total scores." Their conclusion states, "Patients undergoing treatment for knee OA with PRP can be expected to experience improved clinical outcomes when compared with HA." That's the bottom line, but there are other factors such as cost and patient profile that may determine which treatment is the right match. On top of that, we still haven't discovered how the addition of ozone to each of these treatments affects the outcome, and that may just be the most critical factor in determining the treatment of choice.

In 2020, a review[63] was published that compared ozone injections and HA. The review states that "in comparison to corticosteroids, HA injection has been shown to result in more persistent therapeutic effects lasting almost 12 times longer than corticosteroid injections." The conclusion states, "This meta-analysis showed no significant difference between HA and ozone in reducing pain and improving function in patients with knee OA, although the overall results favored HA over ozone." Because the American Academy of Orthopedic Surgeons hasn't signed onto the validity of HA injections, the overall tone of this review is negative toward both treatments. Nevertheless, the study notes that the rapid effect ozone has on reducing pain should be attributed to the anti-inflammatory effect of reducing cytokines and edema.

Why it should be combined. Of most interest to our discussion are the results in one of the studies[64] by Giombini, which included a third group of patients who received both HA and ozone injections. The group that received the combo treatment improved more dramatically than those who received only ozone or only HA. I was shocked to see that ozone therapy was combined with HA injections because neither of these injections are common in the United States. In Italy, where this study originated, it's an area of interest that's being given the attention it deserves.

These results from the above study support the idea that ozone therapy is an incredible complementary treatment when doing joint injections of almost any variety. My contention is not that you should treat degenerative joints, intervertebral disc disease, and more just by injecting ozone, but that if you inject ozone alongside of your standard treatment, you'll improve your chances of success.

Just to add another twist to the narrative, here's a study demonstrating the superiority of HA and PRP in combination as opposed to just HA.[65] Although it didn't compare PRP without HA, it still vividly shows the value of PRP. Instead of concluding that there's no place for HA injections, consider that mild to moderate OA may benefit from HA, but the data seems to indicate a more pronounced effect when done in combination with other injectables, such as PRP and ozone.

What you need.

- HA in vial or single-use syringe
- Needle
- Ozone equipment

The beauty of this injection is that it's simple and requires minimal supplies. Companies like Steris provide products that come in either multi-dose vials or single-use syringes. EverVisc[66] and other products like it have been approved for canine use.

How to administer. Doses will range from 10 to 20 mg with injections every week for a total of three to five injections.[67] Depending on the temperament of the patient and the comfort level of the veterinarian, administering may require sedation or general anesthesia. Once the patient has been sedated, shaved, and prepped, inject the HA and ozone gas into the joint using a 23-27 g needle and syringe. The entire injection can usually be done in less than a minute once you have found the joint capsule.

Because ozone gas expands into the entire treated area and is quickly absorbed into the tissue, it is my opinion that the ozone should be injected first followed by the injection of HA. Alternatively, it is also possible to ozonate the HA prior to injection, similar to PRP. That is the technique used in one study.[68] The question is whether ozonating the HA solution allows the ozone to have as significant of an effect on the treated area. More information is necessary before we will be able to give definitive guidance on this.

Stem cells. Don't believe all the hype. Stem cells may hold a lot of promise, but when we're talking about regenerative injections, they are not the silver bullet. Since the 1980s, an incredible amount of research has been conducted that shows just how important stem cells are to life and to medicine. They are a critical element of our biology, but when it comes to injection therapies, they really haven't shown themselves to be more effective than PRP.

What it is. Stem cells are basically raw material. These special cells can develop into many different types of cells, ranging from muscle to brain tissue. Because of this, they are referred to as undifferentiated cells. Beyond this ability to morph into the type of cell the body needs, they can also perpetually self-renew.

There are two primary classes of stem cells in the body: pluripotent (also known as embryonic) and multipotent (also known as adult or somatic). Pluripotent stem cells can morph into more than 200 different cell types while multipotent stem cells are a bit more limited.

One more distinction I should make is between autologous and allogeneic stem cells. Autologous cells are those that have been harvested from the same patient that will receive them. They came from that patient, and they will be returned to that patient. Allogeneic cells are those that have been harvested from one patient and then injected into another. With allogeneic stem cells, the donor animal's cells are harvested and then processed in a lab where they replicate and have the potential to treat hundreds of other patients.

It's not yet common practice to use allogeneic stem cells, although their use will likely become more commonplace in the future. When a pet goes for a stem cell treatment, the veterinarian will likely be collecting that animal's own multipotent stem cells either from the fat (adipose) or from the bone marrow. These stem cells are commonly referred to as mesenchymal stem cells (MSC). The animal will be placed under general anesthesia while the stem cells are collected. Once collected, the stem cells will be separated out from the rest of the tissue or blood and concentrated down using specialized equipment. They are then reinjected back into the injured area. The entire process typically takes three to four hours, and the pet can go home that same day.

Stem cells work through a few different mechanisms. First, they are anti-inflammatory. Second, they promote angiogenesis, which is the buildup of new blood vessels to improve oxygenation in ischemic or damaged tissue. Third, they are regenerative. Stem cells can send out a signal to recruit other cells to help repair the damage, and they can also morph into the needed tissue to further repair the damage.

Why it should be combined. The combination of ozone and stem cells as a regenerative injection is uncommon. In fact, I had trouble finding a single article that described the combination of ozone therapy with stem cells as an injection. One of the very few I found[69] compared the combination for knee osteoarthritis and showed a more favorable result when combined. Until more information is available, no definitive statement can be made. However, if ozone and stem cells are combined, it would seem prudent to inject ozone prior to the stem cell injection so that the ozone is fully absorbed and has no chance to react with the stem cells. While ozone has been shown to activate platelets when doing PRP treatments, it seems likely that direct interaction with stem cells could have a negative impact on those stem cells.

What you need. As with PRP, you'll need specialized equipment unless you choose to use allogenic stem cells that have been cultivated at a lab. That equipment will include the following:

- Liposuction needle and syringe OR bone marrow extraction kit
- Cell extraction solution
- Centrifuge
- Centrifuge kit

The cost to give a stem cell treatment can exceed $2,000, which means that often the practitioner will charge $4,000–$5,000 for just one treatment. This presents a problem for many because the cost doesn't often outweigh the benefit when compared to some of the other injection or treatment options. I have looked at the studies and talked to a number of veterinarians. The consensus seems to be that, in general, there is no decided benefit to using stem cells over PRP.

How to administer. If using allogenic stem cells, the process is fairly simple because harvesting stem cells is unnecessary. If you are going to be performing an autologous stem cell treatment, it becomes more difficult and time-consuming. Harvesting, preparing, and injecting stem cells require the equipment, knowledge, and skill that only come with practice.

If stem cells are to be collected from the bone marrow, the bone marrow kit will include an introducer needle, stylet, and aspiration cannula. After the animal is put under general anesthesia, the introducer needle is inserted with the stylet via ultrasound guidance. Once it reaches the bone, a small mallet is used to gently tap the needle into the bone. Once at the desired depth, the stylet is removed, and the aspiration cannula is inserted. A syringe is attached, and the marrow is aspirated. The next step is to infuse the stem cells into the centrifuge kit and spin them down. After they have been concentrated, those cells are injected back into the animal.

In animals, it may be easier to gather fat cells from the fatty areas. If stem cells are to be collected from adipose tissue, the kit will include a special syringe, filters, and liposuction cannulas. After the animal is under general anesthesia, the doctor can make an incision and extract the fat using a hemostat and scalpel. Once harvested, there are a few different ways to process the stem cells and separate out the fat so the cells can be injected back into the patient. Some companies advocate using a photoactivator, which stimulates the stem cells prior to injection, but there is little research on this method.

In summary. What we're really trying to do with all of these injection therapies is change the paradigm from reactive, symptom-based medicine to proactive, root cause-based medicine that helps the body repair itself.

Injections for conditions such as arthritis, bursitis, herniated discs, and cruciate injuries are continuing to develop and should be considered as a potential solution prior to surgery or steroids.

In 2017, the *Journal of Orthopaedic Surgery and Research* published a systematic review and meta-analysis of randomized controlled studies.[70] This review compared the results of studies that included saline placebo, HA, ozone, and corticosteroids. The study demonstrated that PRP seems to outshine the other injection types when done by itself.

Another review[71] of injectable therapies compared the literature on OA from corticosteroids, HA, PRP, prolotherapy, stem cells, and genicular nerve blocks. While nerve blocking is outside the scope of this book, the rest of these conditions are relevant. What we notice in both studies is that traditional medicine has nothing on these regenerative injections. In fact, the side effects from corticosteroids should make the choice obvious.

OTHER MODALITIES

"It was about the time that I joined y'all at the first ozone therapy forum and heard about combining acupuncture with ozone," said Dr. Mitch McKee. Dr. McKee continued with the following story:

> She (my client) brought Sabrina in for the first treatment with Sabrina's back legs in a sling. Not really knowing yet how to use the ozone well, I gave 30 ml of ozonated saline on either side of the bladder channel and then did electrical acupuncture. The next day, after we did our first session, the owner walked into the living room and Sabrina was up and walking around. She was not able to use her

back legs one day and then she was up and walking around the next!

Dr. McKee's story highlights the benefit that ozone can have when combined with acupuncture. Each treatment is excellent in its own right, but the effect that they can have together can exceed their individual effect.

A human study[72,] published in 2007 illustrates this proposition. One hundred and twenty patients with low back pain were divided into three groups. The first received electroacupuncture; the second received Danggui (an herb) through an injection point; and the third received ozone through an injection point. The results show "significant differences in the therapeutic effect of the O3 acupoint injection group as compared to the EA group and the Danggui point injection group, but there was no significant difference between the EA group and the Danggui point injection group." The study concluded that ozone acupoint injections are a convenient and highly effective therapy for low back pain.

There are other traditional and nontraditional treatments that work well with ozone therapy. For example, these studies[73,74] discuss the effects of ozone therapy when used to treat the side effects of chemo and radiation. Additionally, it is generally accepted to use ozone therapy alongside various pharmaceuticals without any negative interaction. Because ozone is a nonspecific treatment that induces the body's own healing mechanisms, it tends to play well with all other forms of treatments. To my knowledge, ozone therapy can be utilized with any other treatment without exhibiting any negative side effects. The only potential caveat to this is the use of antioxidants, such as a vitamin C infusion, simultaneously with ozone therapy. If you are going to perform such a treatment, it is best to administer the ozone treatment prior to the antioxidant so the ozone isn't completely exhausted by the antioxidants prior to doing its work. The premise here is somewhat speculative instead of rooted in direct scientific studies. However, until more information is available on this, it would be best practice to follow the above formula.

SUMMARY

Because of its ability to reduce inflammation and promote cellular oxygenation, ozone therapy is a powerful veterinary tool that can help almost every patient. It's not rocket science. Just use ozone therapy alongside the other treatments you're performing, and you're likely to get a better result.

- O3UV is a treatment that combines ozone therapy with UBI. Used together, they have a synergistic effect that produces some pretty incredible results.
- Ozone combined with prolotherapy, PRP, and stem cells for musculoskeletal conditions is a powerful combination.
- Knowing how and when to inject the ozone is crucial to success and can take some practice before feeling comfortable. You need to attend a training class for this.
- Using ozone therapy alongside pharmaceuticals, radiation, and chemo can have beneficial effects and should be a part of your treatment plan for your patients.
- Do ozone therapy at least a few minutes before a High Vitamin C treatment to ensure that the high antioxidant content of the blood doesn't interfere with ozone carrying out its functions.
- Anecdotal evidence indicates that flooding an affected area with ozonated saline and then performing acupuncture or laser therapy over that area potentiates the treatment.

Chapter 7

How to Get Started

*It has become the foundational tool.
A lot of the time it is the reason that
they are coming to me. For my
practice it is THE money maker.*

DR. KATHY BACKUS

If you don't work in a veterinary setting, then this chapter really doesn't apply, and you can skip ahead to the next chapter. For those of you in a veterinary setting who have been doing ozone therapy for years, for those of you who are just getting started, and for those of you who are yet to begin, following the suggestions in this chapter will be crucial to your success.

RETURN ON INVESTMENT (ROI)

If you work in a veterinary practice, then you are part of a business. For a business to thrive, the income must exceed expenses. That's Business 101. Pull that off and you have what's called a profitable business. If I told you that an ozone therapy system and training cost $50,000 (it doesn't) and that you have to replace it every five years (you don't) but you could expect that you would make the $50,000 back over that period of time, would that be a good financial investment? Please answer no. It wouldn't be a good financial investment because you need to bring in more than you spend, and the cost of the equipment up front isn't the only cost that you will incur.

One of the beauties of ozone therapy is that the upfront cost of equipment is the bulk of what you will pay because it generates the medicinal elements necessary to treat the animal. But you can't stop there when considering ROI. The important inputs to consider before implementing ozone therapy in your practice are:

- The upfront cost
- The recurring cost
- The net income generated from offering this treatment
- The residual value of the equipment after the period of time being analyzed

The first three are easy, but the last one may present a question.

Each piece of equipment that you purchase has a lifecycle. On average, how many years can you expect this equipment to last before it is obsolete? For medical equipment, it's not uncommon to have a ten-year lifecycle, whether that means you can expect the device will be damaged, break down, or need to be updated based on technological advances. As you consider ROI, you need to consider all these things and ensure that your company is going to come out on top in the long run. Here's how I break it down in our training class:

Initial Equipment Cost: $8,000

Training Cost: $1,000

Yearly Cost of Supplies: $4,320 (three treatments/day)

Yearly Cost of Labor to Administer: $3,360 (one hr./day)

If you depreciate the device and training across the ten-year period, you would need to recoup $900 each year. We'll add to that the yearly cost of supplies and labor to perform the treatments for a grand total of $8,580 in costs each year. Now, if you charge an average of $55 for each treatment and perform three treatments per day, that means you can count on an additional revenue of $165 each day, $3,300 each month, and $39,600 each year. If you subtract your expenses, you get a yearly net profit of $31,020. Over the lifetime of the equipment, you have a total profit of $310,200. At that rate, you have paid the equipment off within the first year. I don't think I need to tell you that the ROI is through the roof.

While a financial ROI is critical, we haven't even touched on the return you'll get from healthy animals and happy clients. That return truly is priceless and should be a part of the equation. Dr. Shoemaker told me that she has five machines, and she paid each one off in a matter of months:

> Ozone therapy, as I have said many times in my career, is probably the best thing I have added to my practice in my entire career. It is so safe. It is something that can be done by a technician and even an owner (at home) in some instances...It's something that I administer to just about every animal in my clinic because ozone really helps the effectiveness of all my other treatments . . . my ozone machines have all paid for themselves within two to three months of me acquiring them, and I have five. It's really a great investment.

EQUIPMENT

Equipment is a critical topic because the wrong equipment can mean inefficiency, continual maintenance, and even dangerous scenarios. I have talked to a number of people who have decided to bubble ozone into a fluid, but they didn't have equipment specially designed for the task. As a result, they ended up releasing a good amount of ozone into the air, which leads to breathing it in, which leads to irritated lungs. Again, a small amount of ozone here and there isn't going to hurt anyone, but if we are using it day in and day out without the right system, it can really create a problem.

Another scenario I've seen is the use of ozone generators that were designed for air or water purification. When used to create medical-grade ozone, users have no idea what concentration they are going to get or whether the internal components are intended to create ozone that will be used therapeutically. It would seem obvious that this isn't a good idea, but I've run across too many people who considered this a legitimate option.

Beyond these types of issues with equipment, there are the more subtle things to consider as well, such as products that have been specifically designed for animal use or an ozone syringe that won't break down and introduce harmful chemicals into the patient.

Bottom line, if you get your equipment from a conscientious manufacturer (and, of course, I'm a little partial to O3Vets), you can be confident that what you have is perfectly suited for your needs.

Let's now look at the various pieces that make up the ozone system that a veterinarian would need in their clinic. I'm going to separate these components into two categories—ozone generation and accessories.

You'll need the following items to generate medical-grade ozone:

- Ozone Generator
- Oxygen Tank and Medical-Grade Oxygen
- Oxygen Regulator
- Oxygen Tubing

Ozone generator. This is the most important piece of any ozone therapy system. Choosing correctly here will set you up for success, while choosing incorrectly will lead to frustration, wasted time, and wasted money.

There are various types of ozone generators on the market, including designs for industrial uses such as air purification, mold eradication, and water treatment. When we get to medical uses, there are those designed for laboratories, dental use, human use, and animal use. Some of these within the medical category will be used interchangeably, but efficiency, precision, safety, and even efficacy can be compromised depending on the situation. A good example of this is limb bagging. When doing a limb bag treatment, it's both safer and more efficient to have a generator with an active capture. An active capture is basically a pump that sucks the excess ozone out of the bag and through an internal destruct, thereby ensuring no ozone gets into the air.

Before we enumerate the items that make up a good medical ozone generator, you should be aware of the four main ways that ozone is created for commercial and medical use. Those are: corona discharge, cold plasma, UV radiation, and electrolytic. For the right application, each of these has its benefits.

Corona discharge. When a lightning storm takes place, high-voltage electricity rips through our troposphere tearing apart oxygen atoms. Most of those singlet atoms join back together reforming as oxygen (O_2), but a small number of them join together as three oxygen molecules and form ozone (O_3). There are corona discharge generators designed for commercial use and others that have been designed for medical use. Those designed for medical use run medical-grade oxygen past this high voltage and, much like the lightning storm, create ozone. This is currently the best type of ozone generator to use for ozone therapy. It's reliable, precise, safe, budget-friendly, and can be adjusted to generate various concentrations. You may hear people mention "cold corona" or "silent corona" when referring to corona discharge. These are all part of the same basic type of generator. Advances in technology have allowed these generators to improve, reducing the noise and heat needed to generate the ozone, but my experience has been that most manufacturers have adopted the newer standards.

You may hear a lot about whether you should use ceramic, glass, or quartz as the dialectic material where the ozone is produced. The best name for this part of the ozone generator (pictured) is the corona cell, often referred to as the generator or reactor. This part consists of a dialectic barrier, usually made of quartz or ceramic, and an electrode made of some type of conductive material. When high voltage is applied to the electrode and oxygen gas is forced through the corona cell, ozone is produced. While you may hear a lot about whether to use quartz or ceramic, the reality is that this decision is of little importance because they both work well. There are other factors, such as the way the cell is shaped, how the oxygen flows through, what type of electrode material is used, and how big the air gap is that are more important than whether you choose quartz or ceramic for the dialectic barrier.

Hopefully that gives you a quick peek into generator construction, but this isn't the type of information you need to be worrying about, so I'm not going to discuss it any further.

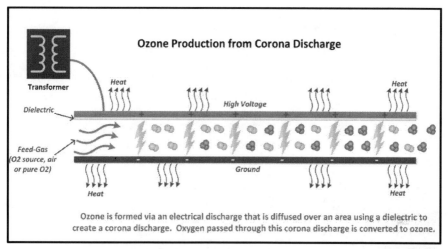

Oxidation Technologies {https://www.oxidationtech.com/downloads/Ozone_Production/Ozone_Generated_by_Corona_Discharge.png}

Cold plasma. Plasma is a fourth state of matter after solids, fluids, and gases. It is an ionized, electrically conductive, gaseous material. There is a lot of confusion and misinformation surrounding the definition of cold plasma ozone generators.

I have been in this industry for more than ten years, and I was never quite sure what a cold plasma ozone generator really was. Reading blogs and readily available information on the internet led to more confusion. For example, some sites say that if you use pure oxygen to create the ozone, your generator should be considered cold plasma. Others say that if you use oxygen, a dialectic barrier, and the electrodes are enclosed in glass, it is a plasma generator. It wasn't until I really dug in and started reading the scientific studies that I was able to grasp what is really going on here. It comes down to the fact that ozone generators using corona discharge also ionize atoms and generate a field of plasma.[75] It is true that a dialectic barrier like quartz or ceramic will assist in the production of plasma, so it could be said that this technology is a cold plasma generator, or it could be said that it is a corona discharge generator. Both of these statements would be true, but the use of the term "cold plasma" has often been manipulated by a marketing department instead of used as a scientific term by engineering. The materials used, the gas introduced, and the way the generator is designed all play a role in whether a smaller or larger plasma field is created. However, the goal of an ozone generator is NOT to make plasma but to generate ozone.[76]

The important thing to pay attention to when purchasing an ozone generator is not whether it's cold plasma or corona discharge, but if it meets the criteria set forth in the list that that starts in a couple of paragraphs, but first let's look at two more types of ozone generators.

UV radiation. In our atmosphere, UV rays from the sun come into contact with oxygen to make ozone. This constitutes our ozone layer, which effectively blocks the UV-C rays from reaching the Earth's surface. In a generator that uses UV light, ambient air flows past UV lamps to generate ozone. It's the least efficient way to produce ozone, but the process can be great for air purifiers. These generators are not recommended for ozone therapy.

Electrolytic. These generators rely solely on the oxygen within water to produce ozone. This method eliminates the need for a separate oxygen source and is often used in pharmaceutical, cosmetic, and personal care product markets that need high purity water. It is not a good type of ozone generator for ozone therapy unless it is being used solely to create ozonated fluids.

Choosing your generator. There are a few criteria that should be at the top of your list when shopping for an ozone generator.

Safety. If we do harm in the process of treating a patient, then the good we do can be overshadowed by the undesirable side effects. For example, if we are using an ozone generator that doesn't have an auto shut off feature to stop producing ozone if no syringe is connected, then we can inadvertently create ozone that enters the room and is breathed in by the patient and the user. Features such as luer-lock connections, auto shut off, and live concentration analysis all make a device safer for the patient and the user. We'll get into some of these below.

Ozone resistant parts. An ozone generator cannot be manufactured with parts that corrode and disintegrate when they come into contact with ozone. Make sense? I feel a bit ridiculous making that statement, but I suppose it's possible to find a manufacturer who uses the wrong types of materials. How will you know? About a year into using the machine, you'll notice that it doesn't work like it used to. There is corrosion or a constant smell of ozone when you're generating it. Really, there's no way to know before this happens, so make sure to choose a company with a good reputation when purchasing an ozone generator.

A lot has been written about the material used for the reactor—the part of the ozone generator where ozone is produced. Should it be a single piece of quartz glass? Is ceramic okay? What about stainless steel? It seems as if quartz glass and ceramic are the materials of choice, but good data that sets one apart from the other is difficult to come by. Most of the noise out there is from manufacturers who want you to buy their product. Don't get caught up in the crossfire of information from manufacturers.

Flow rate. A generator that allows the user to finish a daily treatment in five minutes as opposed to ten minutes will save about 20 hours of time each year. Time is money, and most of us are short on both. A generator that can produce a high concentration (i.e., 50 µg/ml) and a high flow rate (i.e., 1/2 LPM) at the same time is going to get the job done faster.

Concentration. In medical ozone it's most common to use concentrations under 50 µg/ml, but when ozonating a fluid or limb bagging, it can be helpful to have concentrations of up to 80 µg/ml. Ensuring that the ozone generator produces ozone at these higher levels will mean that you'll always have the concentration you need. Ideally, you'll purchase a generator that's able to produce between 1-80 µg/ml. Anything above 80 µg/ml is unnecessary.

Modes. Having a variety of modes is helpful. For example, when you want to ozonate a fluid or fill a limb bag, it's important to have a continuous flow mode that allows you to produce ozone for a set amount of time and then automatically shut off. A mode that will allow you to simply set the concentration and then automatically fill a syringe makes ozone injections a snap. Modes will make the treatments faster, easier, and more efficient.

Medical connections. The most common connection used for attaching a syringe to the generator is the Luer-lock connection. This lock ensures a universal, secure fit every time you connect a tube or syringe to your generator. Other connection types can work but are more cumbersome and less secure. Having a push connector that securely connects the oxygen tubing to the generator and regulator is also very nice.

Live concentration analysis. There are three main ways to calculate the concentration output on an ozone generator. The most common is for the manufacturer to design the generator to their own specifications and then apply a chart onto the generator that indicates the concentration depending on the oxygen flow speed (i.e., 1/4 LPM) and the amount of voltage applied to the reactor. If the voltage can be adjusted, it's usually via a knob on the front of the generator that has a setting between 1 and 10. Keep in mind that some generators have no voltage adjustment, and the only thing that can be adjusted is the oxygen flow speed.

The second way to calculate the concentration is through software built into the device that utilizes a mathematical algorithm. These types of generators always have an interface that allows the user to select the desired concentration. The generator will then produce the selected concentration.

The third way to calculate the concentration is with a spectrophotometer. This special device is built into the generator and uses UV light to measure ozone through analyzing the percentage of light absorbed by the ozone.

All three methods can be effective if the ozone generator has been properly designed, but the latter is the most desirable. Having a spectrophotometer that gives live concentration analysis will increase the cost of the generator but will also provide peace of mind that you are producing the proper concentration for the patient you are treating.

Integrated destruct. A destruct is usually a short stainless-steel tube containing a dark granular form of manganese dioxide catalyst. A destruct can be built into the generator and have a Luer-lock connection to easily connect a syringe or other accessory. When the ozone flows through this material, it converts back to oxygen making it safe to breathe. There are various kinds of this material, but the best is a formula that includes copper oxide, ensuring that it won't be consumed by ozone and thereby providing a long lifetime.

Keep in mind that the enemy of any of these catalyst materials is moisture, so it's vital that you keep any fluids out of the destruct. If you ever find that your destruct isn't working properly, it's likely because it has become moist from humidity or fluid ingress.

Information readout. During or after the ozone production phase, you'll want to know just how much ozone was produced. This can be especially helpful when filling a bag for rectal insufflation. Because an insufflation bag (unlike a syringe) is able to expand, it is impossible to know just how much ozone is in the bag unless you have an information readout that gives you this data. An information readout can also provide other information, such as when calibration is necessary, whether a specific error is causing the device to malfunction, and so on.

Warranty and servicing. Like any device, ozone generators can have problems. If you find a company that offers long warranties and fast, local service, it's well worth the extra cost.

Beware of the "reactor" or "electrode" warranty, which only covers one part of the ozone generator. (I find the best term for this part is "reactor" because it's where the oxygen and high voltage react to create ozone.) This is a part that likely will never cause any problems and, therefore, is easy to guarantee. However, a long-term warranty on the entire generator is a wonderful indication of quality and company commitment to the product.

Training and support. Although not a physical piece of the generator, training and support are two of the most important issues when it comes to purchasing ozone therapy equipment.

Have you ever made a purchase just to have it sit in a closet collecting dust? The ozone generator is only as good as the professional punching its buttons, and that professional won't be prepared to fully utilize ozone therapy to its full potential unless they are trained. So, when purchasing, don't just look at features or price. Make sure that the company you purchase from has a good reputation for training and supporting their clients along the way. This support should include not only equipment setup and operation but also training on how to administer the treatments, what to charge, how ozone therapy works, what it's indicated for, etc.

OXYGEN

Oxygen is vital to the production of medical-grade ozone. Here is a breakdown of the various oxygen purity levels.

The air we breathe	21%
An oxygen concentrator	90-95%
Industrial-grade oxygen	99.5%
Medical-grade oxygen	99.5%
Food-grade oxygen	99.9%
Ultra-high purity grade	99.993%
Research-grade oxygen	99.999%

Medical-grade oxygen is the oxygen most commonly used for ozone therapy, and it provides high purity ozone. As you will notice in the chart above, industrial-grade oxygen is the same purity as medical-grade, but don't let that fool you. There is a difference between them. The difference comes down to the fact that the oxygen tanks used for industrial oxygen are not checked for purity like their counterparts in the medical field.

Because of this, it is possible that impurities exist within the tank, which could result in unwanted gases. To avoid the slight chance of any impurities, best practice is to use medical-grade oxygen to feed your ozone generator. The only consideration with this choice is that you'll need a medical prescription or a medical license to rent or purchase medical oxygen. For a veterinarian, this shouldn't be any problem, but if you're not a doctor, you will need to get a prescription or just go with the industrial oxygen tank.

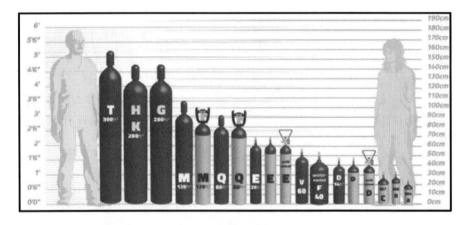

Tank size is another consideration. Medical oxygen tanks start at an M2, which will fit in a purse, and go up to a T tank, which stands over five feet tall. Here in the United States, most medical tanks are made from aluminum and have the brushed steel look with a green top. The exception to this comes when you get up to about 7,000 liters. Most of the time these larger tanks are made from a heavy steel and are painted green.

So which tank sizes are best for ozone therapy? The answer depends on whether you're a mobile, small animal, or a large animal vet. If you have an anesthesia machine, you probably already have large H or K tanks. That's great, but you'll either need a tank dedicated to ozone or you'll need to tap into your existing oxygen supply lines with the proper adaptors to feed your ozone generator. If you choose to use a tank, I find that it's most common for a veterinary clinic to use an E tank or a D tank, but I recommend having more than one on hand. If you are a large animal or mobile vet, you'll also want to have a small tank that's easy to carry with you. Your best bet is the M6 tank. Keep in mind that it will need to be filled more frequently because it is small.

Once you decide on your oxygen tank, you'll need to make sure that you purchase the corresponding oxygen regulator. All medical tanks up to the E size use a CGA 870 style regulator. For tanks larger than the E tank, you'll need to get a CGA 540 style regulator.

As an aside, a transfill hose allows you to connect two oxygen tanks and then transfer oxygen from one tank to the other. Purchasing a transfill hose will allow you to fill a small tank from a large tank. This can be helpful if you don't want to mess with calling the oxygen company every time you need to fill a smaller tank. Keep in mind that the transfill hose allows oxygen to flow from the tank with the greater pressure to the tank with the lesser pressure. So, for example, if your small M6 tank has 1,000 psi and your large K tank has 900 psi, you'll actually transfer oxygen from the smaller tank to the larger tank. For this refill to work, the larger tank must always have a good deal more pressure than the small tank.

I have been asked many times about using an oxygen concentrator to produce ozone. In the past, I imported equipment from Professor Eugeny Nazarov of the Ukraine. In Ukraine and Russia, oxygen concentrators are commonly used to feed ozone generators. It is especially common for continuous flow applications such as the ozonation of fluids or limb bagging. My position is to use medical-grade oxygen and not fuss with an oxygen concentrator. The first problem with an oxygen concentrator is that some generators simply won't work with one because it won't supply enough pressure. With other generators, the ozone concentration will be different than what you think you're getting. The final concern is production of secondary gases that may be harmful. Because we are introducing a certain percentage of nitrogen into the ozone generator instead of pure oxygen, there is the potential for creating other harmful chemical compounds that are then introduced into the patient. For these reasons, I don't recommend the use of an oxygen concentrator.

DECIDING ON ACCESSORIES

The generator usually comes with everything you need to generate ozone, but you'll also need to purchase accessories that will allow you to apply ozone to the patient in the appropriate ways. Since we've already walked through the various administration methods in chapter four, we don't need to reiterate that information. What you need to know now is what items you'll need for each ozone administration method. Let's take a look.

Fluid bubbler. Fluid bubblers come in different sizes and shapes, but their purpose is simple. If you want to saturate a fluid with ozone so that you can use it therapeutically, you'll need a fluid bubbler. This is one of the pieces I consider essential for every ozone therapy system. As a veterinarian, you'll want a bubbler that holds at least 1,000 ml and has an integrated destruct. It's also very helpful if it can be attached to an IV pole for ease of use. For use at home, a 500 ml bubbler is sufficient.

Fluid jars. Unless kept in a refrigerator and stored in an ozone resistant jar, ozonated fluids will break down very quickly. With a special jar and ozone resistant lids, you can store fluids in the refrigerator for up to three days. This is especially helpful if you want to send this home with your clients so they can benefit from the use of fluid while not in the clinic.

Rectal insufflation kit. Ozone resistant rectal catheters, syringes, and insufflation bags are important, and like the bubbler, they are an essential part of your ozone therapy system. Ozone resistant syringes can usually hold up to 60 ml while the insufflation bags can hold up to 750 ml. The bags can be used for large dogs or large animals when necessary. These bags are also commonly used for humans when they practice these treatments on themselves.

Limb bag kit. The limb bag kit is designed to perform ozone gas treatments on the leg of an animal. It is commonly used for wounds, ulcers, and surgery sites. This kit is made up of the different pieces you'll need to safely administer ozone in the clinic. Proper technique is extremely important when you are doing this treatment, so having the proper pieces will set you up for success.

Oil bubbler. Having an oil bubbler is NOT so that you can make your own oils to use in the clinic. The bubbling of ozone through oil for long periods of time can create a fire hazard. Beyond that, the process is long, arduous, and needs the proper equipment to ensure purity in the oil while keeping the oil at proper temperatures. Bubbling ozone through oil changes the oil from ozone gas to ozonides and peroxides, many of which are trapped in the oil itself. Once the oil has been sufficiently saturated, an ozonide vapor is released from the oil and can be safely breathed. This is often used for respiratory conditions.

Ear insufflation cups. These cups can be attached to the oil bubbler to allow the ozonide vapor to sift into the ear canal to treat infections. They can also be connected directly to the ozone generator so that ozone gas can be applied directly to the ears.

Inhalation mask. Like the ear insufflation cups, an inhalation mask can be connected to the oil bubbler to allow a patient to breathe the ozonide vapor. It is most commonly used for respiratory conditions. By way of disclaimer, this method has anecdotal evidence of efficacy but does not yet have the backing of scientific studies.

Topicals. Ozone oils, creams, gels, sprays, and shampoos can be used topically to treat skin conditions including autoimmune and infectious. These are especially helpful to send home with clients after their pet has received an ozone treatment in the clinic. The active ingredient in all of these topical products is going to be some sort of ozonated oil. When deciding on which topical product is best, I tend to lean toward one of the topicals that has been specially formulated to absorb into the skin. The oils by themselves tend to be a little messy and smelly, but their effectiveness is unquestionable.

TRAINING

Someday ozone therapy will be taught in veterinary schools across the country and around the world, but as of now, the entire educational process will happen after you've graduated from veterinary school.

O3Vets offers a veterinary training course that can be completed in a few days and equips a veterinarian with the basics to understand and administer ozone therapy in the clinic. There are also webinars, protocol videos, equipment how-to videos, testimonials, and more available on O3Vets' YouTube channel at www.youtube.com/o3vets as well as an online training course available at www.vetozonetraining.com.

THE ROLL-OUT PLAN

Before Dr. Andrea Carlson even had the equipment, she began telling clients about ozone therapy and how she was going to be adding it to her practice. Soon enough, she had a waiting list of clients excited about their pets being one of the first to receive an ozone therapy treatment at her clinic in Merrillville, Indiana. Dr. Carlson used that excitement to generate momentum, which led to greater acceptance of the treatment as well as a quick ROI.

At a recent veterinary ozone therapy training class, Dr. Alton Raymond told us about a novel idea he had that led to some incredible testimonies and an increase of over $2,000 a month in additional revenue for his clinic. He decided that he would keep his clinic open for a few hours after closing and provide ozone therapy treatments to patients during that window. A few technicians stay late to manage these customers and administer the treatments. The beauty of this technique is not only the additional revenue but also the conversation that happens among clients. "These clients hang out together in the waiting room discussing ozone therapy and how it has benefited their pet," said Dr. Raymond. "They end up selling the treatment to other clients for me!"

SUMMARY

Whether you use either technique above, you must have a plan for how you intend to use ozone therapy and how you intend to get clients interested in paying for the treatment. Here are several keys to successfully integrating ozone therapy into your practice:

1. Decide on where you will put your "ozonation station" and purchase the proper equipment
2. Get training for you and your staff
3. Prepare or purchase marketing materials for your clients
4. Set pricing, upsells, and treatment package plans
5. Create a kickoff event at your clinic
6. Get continuing education to become a better ozone therapist

Many veterinarians stop after one and a half steps. They get the equipment and then get just enough training to get started but don't put in the time to fully prepare. If you follow the formula above, you will be set up nicely for success. Not cutting corners in the beginning will lead to a much better ROI in the end.

Chapter 8

Putting It All Together

*I think ozone therapy is a crucial part
of the 21st-century veterinary clinic.*

DR. ALLEN SCHOEN

If you feel confident that you know the information in this book, you can skip this chapter and use it as a resource down the road. If you're just picking up this book and are tempted to skip all the previous chapters, you are making a mistake. I understand that time is our most precious commodity, and it can be difficult to set aside time to slow down and read, but I want to let you in on a little secret: reading this book from cover to cover will take the average reader less than three hours. That's right, less time than it takes me to watch the Detroit Lions lose a football game on a Sunday afternoon. Learning takes time.

INTRODUCTION

It starts with a paradigm shift. Embracing ozone therapy doesn't have to mean that you understand treating disease outside of the context of drugs and surgery, but to utilize ozone to its full potential does mean just that. It shouldn't be relegated to the use of ozonated fluids in the surgery room or the combination of ozone with PRP for musculoskeletal issues. I've said this before, but it's important to remember that ozone therapy is a powerful veterinary tool that can help almost every patient because of its ability to reduce inflammation and promote cellular oxygenation.

CHAPTER 1 - HOW OXYGEN DEFICIENCY AND INFLAMMATION ARE KILLING OUR ANIMALS

The role of oxidative stress and chronic inflammation in disease is undeniable. Poor oxygen utilization on a cellular level is a sure indicator that dysregulation is occurring. As we learned, the specific dysregulation that occurs in many chronic illnesses is the overproduction of immune cells and the underproduction of antioxidants, which leads to oxidative stress and inflammation. It's precisely at this point that ozone therapy plays a critical role.

CHAPTER 2 – OZONE AS A THERAPY... REALLY?

When a treatment comes along that isn't a drug, it is almost always met with skepticism and rejection. That's because we have a highly developed, fiercely protected health system. Pharmaceutical companies will do almost anything to keep the status quo because they have a really good thing going. Why would you jeopardize a near monopoly on educational institutions, insurance companies, and hospitals? Plus, pharmaceuticals have proven to be helpful in many instances. It's really a win-win . . . at times. Something like ozone therapy is a win for patients who want to get better without side effects, but it's a loss for pharmaceutical companies who want to maintain profits.

It's incumbent upon companies like O3Vets, institutions like the University of Bari Aldo Moro in Italy, and veterinarians like Dr. Margo Roman to help turn the tide in favor of these types of treatments.

CHAPTER 3 – HOW IT WORKS

Although we don't fully understand the mechanism of action, ongoing research has helped clarify some things for us that are now beyond question. For example, we now understand that ozone's antimicrobial capabilities are not at the center of its mechanism of action for most disease processes. We now clearly see that ozone works to reduce inflammation while improving cellular oxygenation. We also know that it helps regulate the production of immune cells, which is attributed to ozone acting as a redox signaling molecule.

Within medicine, a full-orbed understanding of the mechanism is almost impossible for any treatment because of the complexity of the body's systems. However, we've come a long way in understanding ozone therapy and continue to press toward an even greater and more nuanced understanding.

CHAPTER 4 – HOW TO ADMINISTER OZONE

Most medical treatments can only be administered in only one way. In this book, we discussed sixteen, yes, sixteen ways that ozone therapy can be administered. Each of these ways falls under the category of systemic or local administration. An example of systemic administration is Major Autohemotherapy. An example of local administration is intra-articular injections. The use of ozonated oils, ozonated fluids, insufflations, injections, infusion of ozone and blood, and inhalation of ozonides are all legitimate ways to administer ozone therapy. This increases the value of the therapy because it increases the number of patients that can benefit from it. Got surgery scheduled? Make sure your ozonated fluids are charged. Have a derm patient coming in? Send them home with ozonated cream. What about the lymphoma case you're seeing? Administering O3UV is a great option.

You may never use all the ozone administration methods in your practice, but it's good to realize that you can always learn and expand on what you are currently doing. Start with one or two of the most basic methods and move up from there.

CHAPTER 5 – CONDITIONS AND HOW TO TREAT THEM

The variety of administration methods is part of what makes ozone therapy so valuable, but when you pair that with how it works to decrease inflammation and improve cellular oxygen, it just makes sense to use ozone therapy in any number of cases.

When I am asked what conditions ozone therapy should be used to treat, it's tough to answer. The *Madrid Declaration on Ozone Therapy* attempts to answer this question by splitting the conditions into three levels. **Level A** includes conditions that have a good scientific basis and include KOA, diabetic foot ulcers, spinal diseases, and proctitis. **Level B** includes conditions that have fair scientific evidence and include orthopedic and traumatology issues, as well as some infections and autoimmune diseases. **Level C** includes conditions that have fair but not enough scientific evidence (when the guide was published in 2020) to convincingly demonstrate safety and efficacy. These conditions include various auto-immune conditions such as Crohn's, MS, psoriasis, and other conditions like chronic kidney failure, liver diseases, respiratory diseases, and more.

While we strive to have undeniable scientific proof that ozone therapy works for everything we treat, it's impossible to provide the level of evidence necessary for each condition without countless hours and millions of dollars in funding. So rather than use the list in the *Madrid Declaration on Ozone Therapy*, I encourage people to use it based on the mechanism of action as well as precedence.

Because of its ability to reduce inflammation and promote cellular oxygenation, ozone therapy is a powerful veterinary tool that can help almost every patient. In most cases, ozone therapy is a nonspecific treatment that helps the body heal itself. This is why it can be successfully implemented as a primary or adjunct treatment for so many different disease processes.

CHAPTER 6 - THE MULTIMODAL APPROACH: COMBINING OZONE WITH OTHER TREATMENTS

I watched a comedian, Brian Regan, talk about how cranberry juice was getting into all the other juices. He proceeded to say, "What do you have, apples? Why don't you put some cranberries in them, call it cranapple; we'll go 50/50. What do you have, grapes? How 'bout crangrape? What do you got, mangos? What about cranmango?" Sometimes I feel like that cranberry salesman who's getting into all the other juices when it comes to ozone therapy, but ozone therapy is a perfect complement to many different treatments because of how it works. I know we could identify more, but understanding how ozone therapy can be combined with UV irradiation and a variety of injection therapies is my primary purpose. I'll briefly mention a couple other treatments, including acupuncture and chemo/radiation.

O3UV is the combination of ozone therapy with UBI. A small amount of blood is withdrawn and treated with ozone and UV light before being reinfused to the patient. There are numerous studies that demonstrate that this combination can be an even more effective way to treat a patient than ozone therapy alone.

You should also take note that the use of ozone with PRP, prolotherapy, and stem cells can lead to a better outcome for these injection therapies. There's quite a bit of research showing that this is a valid way to treat a variety of musculoskeletal conditions.

To my knowledge, there really isn't a treatment or drug that can't be used in conjunction with ozone therapy, but we need more scientific information to create a strong basis for more combination treatments.

CHAPTER 7 – HOW TO GET STARTED

What good is this book unless you pick up the treatment and use it? My purpose is to be intensely practical so that you and your patients or pets can benefit from this treatment.

To be successful, the first thing you need to be convinced of is that there's either a monetary and/or health benefit that exceeds the cost of the equipment. Ask one of the many veterinarians and pet owners who I have personally worked with, and you'll get an unequivocal and immediate answer affirming the value of ozone therapy. Once you are convinced of that, it's a matter of understanding what equipment and training you will need. If you already have equipment, then you need to be trained. If you are already trained, then it may be that you can benefit from more advanced training or from participating in the yearly International Veterinary Ozone Therapy Summit that unites veterinarians from around the world to discuss the advances in veterinary ozone therapy.

A FINAL WORD

Keeping this book on the shelf as a guide is a wonderful idea, but I would also ask you to join us in spreading the word. Consider getting another copy to provide to a friend or colleague and help us bring ozone therapy to the masses. When we find something this good, kindness and compassion compel us to share it. There are others out there suffering who could benefit from ozone therapy, and our common goal is to see them restored to health. So, here's my challenge to you: find one person to share this book with, and let's start an ozone therapy revolution!

Appendix I

A Note on Anticoagulants

Choosing the right anticoagulant shouldn't be a difficult process for veterinarians. With ozone therapy, we use anticoagulants when we do MAHT, mAHT, and with combination treatments like O3UV.

The following is a list of the various injectable anticoagulants that you can use (I find that most veterinarians use heparin):

- Heparin
- Ethylenediaminetetraacetic acid (EDTA)
- Acid citrate dextrose (ACD)—consists of sodium citrate, citric acid, dextrose, and distilled water
- Citrate-phosphate-dextrose-adenine (CPDA-1)—one of the most popular anticoagulants in human and veterinary transfusion medicine
- Iloprost
- Rivaroxaban
- Apixaban

Once you have chosen the anticoagulant that you believe will best suit your needs, you must then determine the dose that you intend to use. With heparin, it's common to use 50 units per 1 ml of blood. Since most vials of heparin have 10,000 units per ml, you'll usually end up using less than a tenth of an ml per treatment.

Appendix II

How to Administer Ozone at Home

You're probably here because you have a pet who is suffering. You'll want to visit www.o3pets.com for more information. Recognize that an investment in ozone therapy equipment and the knowledge that you'll need are going to be a wonderful addition to helping your pet heal, but it's more than that. You can use this treatment for years to come for yourself and any pet you'll have. This treatment is something that should be in every home as an essential part of the family's medical care.

I personally have an ozone generator, the accessories, and the topical ozone products. I use ozone-infused toothpaste every day to maintain good oral health, and I keep Hydrogel 15% on hand for anything more serious. I have ozonated shampoo to care for the scalp, reduce dandruff, and oxygenate. I also have ozonated ear drops for ear infections. Honesto3 (www.honesto3.com) carries Pet Liniment 10% and Lipogel 15% for first-aid, rashes, and more. With all these topicals and the ozone therapy equipment, I feel like we can take on whatever presents itself with more confidence.

So, let's talk about the steps to using ozone therapy at home.

VETERINARY OVERSIGHT

The first non-negotiable is putting yourself under the care and direction of a licensed veterinarian who has the right to prescribe this treatment for your pet in the state or province where you live. Legally, the government cannot stop you from treating your own animals, but wisdom would dictate that you consult with a professional who understands biology, medicine, and disease to effectively prescribe the proper treatments and/or medications. Also, if you choose to use medical-grade oxygen, you'll need to obtain a prescription from a veterinarian to purchase the oxygen.

EQUIPMENT

When it comes to at-home treatments, a basic ozone generator and a few accessories are sufficient. Here's what you should look for:

- A simple, reliable, medical ozone generator
- Supplies for rectal insufflation, including an ozone syringe and rectal catheters
- A fluid bubbler and destruct

You should be able to purchase everything you need for around $1,000, and it should last for many years. If you want a portable setup that you can wheel around, O3Vets sells a cart that can hold all your ozone supplies in one place and be easily moved around the house.

TRAINING

Don't just buy the equipment from a company that doesn't offer support and training. Equipment is no good if you don't have the skill and confidence to use it. It's also no good if you have a scare and then stop using it. You should have . . . no, you NEED a company by your side that will stand by its products and guide you to success. The training shouldn't merely be answering a few questions but an actual dedicated time, whether that's an hour or ten hours, to get you prepared to take on the world with ozone therapy. There are dangers, concerns, and pitfalls that need to be expertly navigated to deliver successful results. Don't go it alone. No one needs to be a hero here, just wise. I have put together the Pet Ozone Academy, which will give you all the training you need to safely and successfully carry this out under the oversight of your veterinarian. You can contact O3Vets for more information.

OXYGEN

Only veterinarians or medical doctors can prescribe medical-grade oxygen, so you need to make a choice. Do you use an industrial oxygen tank or a medical tank? If you need more instruction on this, please check out the section on oxygen in chapter 7. Best practice would be to obtain a medical oxygen tank from a local medical oxygen supply company and then exchange it whenever you need more oxygen. Most commonly, a D tank will suffice and last for three to six months, depending on how many treatments you are doing and whether you are ozonating fluids often. If you choose to go with an industrial tank, a 20 cubic-foot tank will work.

TAKE THE LEAP

Once you have your equipment and you've been properly instructed, you need to step out in confidence and start treating. Don't be afraid. You have a team behind you who will help support and guide you. From your veterinarian to the company you chose to provide your equipment, you'll be prepared to deal with whatever comes.

Appendix III

Industrial Uses of Ozone

Depending on the situation, ozone generators that are larger than a car or smaller than a purse can be used to bring about purification, remediation, and a return to a cleaner Earth. Let's look at just a few ways that ozone is used every day in an environmentally friendly way to make our lives cleaner and healthier.

WATER DISINFECTION

Byproducts from pharmaceutical, textile, automotive, and other industries lead to contaminated water that must be treated. This water can carry contaminants such as cyanides, sanitary waste, phenols, dyes, and more.[77]

There are many advantages that ozone provides over UV or chlorine treatment, such as clearer water and a complete lack of harmful residuals. The residuals that are found after use of chlorine are called disinfection byproducts (DBP), and they have been shown to negatively impact both aquatic and human life. By comparison, using ozone to disinfect water truly is an economical and eco-friendly method. Because ozone breaks down quickly once it contacts organic material, there is no risk of negatively impacting aquaculture once the water is routed into nearby rivers.

ODOR TREATMENT

Floods and fires can cause serious damage that leaves significant odors behind. Structures that are not properly remediated will continue to depredate due to mold, bacteria, and fungus that were not dealt with. Ozone is the strongest oxidant that doesn't leave residual behind. At the right concentrations, it breaks down these organic compounds. This process converts ozone back to oxygen, leaving the area clean and safe. Because high levels of ozone will likely be needed, high-output generators must be used, and the entire area must be evacuated. In the initial phase of the remediation, the levels of ozone will be quite low because of all the impurities in the air and surfaces, but as time goes on and those impurities are reduced, the ozone levels will rise. Often, ozone saturation levels will top out at about 10 ppm in this type of setting. Air blowers will be required to circulate the ozone which will tend to sink to the floor because it is heavier than air. This entire process will last at least a couple of hours in an average room and possibly up to an entire day depending on the severity. Ozone can be a fantastic choice for remediating odors caused by smoke, mold, fungus, or other toxins.[78]

FACILITY AND EQUIPMENT SANITATION

Ozone has been used for years to sanitize equipment and facilities from homes to hospitals. In a recent study[79], the use of humidifiers along with ozone generators was demonstrated to effectively disinfect all surfaces in a room without using any consumables.

Ozone by itself isn't going to be as effective against certain respiratory viruses like the one in this study, but when high humidity is introduced into the room via a humidifier, the effectiveness is complete. Not only that, but once the ozone breaks down, there are no potentially harmful residues left behind.

FOOD PRESERVATION

The decontamination of food and beverages with microorganisms along the processing journey is a key to producing high-quality products. Ozone can play a role in the decontamination process in fruits, vegetables, meat, spices, and beverages. The ozone decontamination process also extends shelf-life.[80]

In 1982, ozone was approved as generally recognized as safe (GRAS) and then approved by the FDA in 2001. It is also approved as organic by the National Organic Program's Final Rule.[81]

Ozone can be applied directly to food or bubbled into a beverage, and it is also useful to clean the surfaces that come into contact with the food as well as the water used to wash it.

From industrial-size solutions to a countertop model that sits by your sink at home, ozone equipment can be a part of providing healthy food that tastes good and stays fresh longer.[82]

AIR PURIFICATION

Much has been made of air purifiers that put out low levels of ozone in a home or office setting. The general consensus is that they should never be used. It's my opinion that every home should have an air purifier that has the option to produce ozone. Users should be judicious when they use the generator, but it's foolish to write ozone generators off simply because they can be misused. A 2017 study found that, at low concentrations, rats (which are very sensitive to ozone) were unharmed when air purifiers putting out .05 ppm were used 24 hours per day for 28 days.[83] This is a VERY low level of ozone, but it demonstrates that, at the very least, there are levels that are appropriate and may help sanitize an area.

So when should we consider using ozone air purifiers and which ones should we use? My recommendation is to find a generator that can be adjusted to put out a higher or lower concentration. It should also have an auto-off capacity so that if you are going to be out of the house for a day, you could run the generator for a few hours before it automatically shuts off. This allows time for the ozone that's produced to do its job and revert back to oxygen.

SOIL REMEDIATION

Inorganic contaminants such as diesel fuel, pesticides, and a variety of VOCs can remain in the soil for decades, impervious to breakdown by microorganisms. Over a period of a few weeks, ozone can dissolve hydrocarbons, leading to the reduction of up to 99% of contaminants. This method can be very beneficial, especially when the location of the soil makes it impossible to replace.

Why Medical Ozone Therapy? Why Microbiome Restorative Therapy (MBRT)? Now and Together

Margo Roman, DVM, CVA, COT, CPT, FAAO

www.mashvet.com

A worldwide study published in 2022 shows that, in 2019, there were 4,950,000 deaths associated with antimicrobial resistance (AMR).[84] For too many years, indiscriminate use of antibiotics, pesticides, herbicides, drugs, and chemicals have destroyed and altered the internal ecosystems of humans and animals. It is crucial that we protect the microbiome and simultaneously stop infection and support the immune system. Stewarding medicine well means giving bodies a healthier way to reduce infection and inflammation to allow the natural healing process.

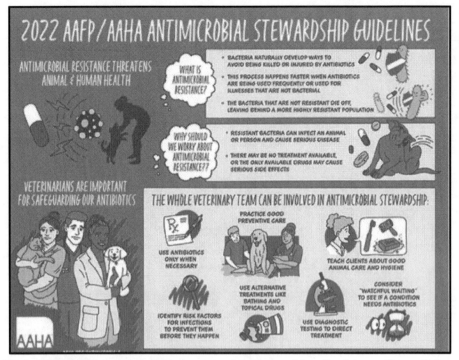

Emily Mills (2002) AAFP/AAHA Antimicrobial Stewardship Guidelines. { https://flavor-graphics.com/about/}

In July 2022, the AVMA, AAHA, and AAFP joined together to bring important changes to the way we use antimicrobials. There are alternatives, and we need to understand how these alternatives will help us do a better job caring for our patients and protecting people from one of the deadliest killers on earth. There are many alternatives that can aid in stopping an infection. Getting some training and exposure to good techniques will be helpful to every veterinarian's practice. Some of these treatment alternatives include:

- Herbs
- Medical ozone
- Laser
- UBI

- Homeopathy
- Photobiomodulation
- Manuka honey

Even simple things like extensive soaking and flushing in warm water, sea salt, and Epsom salts have some value. We must fight the urge to immediately prescribe an antibiotic just because it's the way we do things.

For over 25 years, I haven't used antibiotics for dentals, even with dogs that have heart conditions. Using homeopathics like arnica, silicia, calendula, and hypericum reduces pain and stops infections. Herbal mixtures with echinacea and green tea are also helpful. But the best treatment I have used to treat infections during my career is ozone therapy.

Used by human biological dentists around the world, it helps us solve difficult problems without reaching for antibiotics. Ozone therapy can be used for pain, infection, flushing of debris from the pockets, reducing the infected biofilm, and oxygenating gums, which expedites healing. It also eliminates the need to culture out every pocket, root, and area of gingivitis since ozone destroys bacteria indiscriminately. If bacteria isn't tested to determine what type it is, you could be prescribing an ineffective antibiotic. Again, ozone eliminates that problem.

Microbiome has become the new frontier in medicine. Until the year 2000, we never thought it was important in keeping people and animals healthy. Since 80% of the immune system comes from the gut microbes, it is crucial that we keep this organ system in balance and all species in a symbiotic relationship. Considered the second brain, so much information needs to originate from this vital system. We need to protect the microbes in the mouth as well as the microbes in the gut. Using ozone to remove biofilm in those areas will help to perform MBRT without an antibiotic.

Prior to performing MBRT, I use an ozone concentration of approximately 35 µg/ml to disrupt the biofilm. I infuse ozone gas into the colon and place it as far cranial up the descending colon toward the transverse colon. Once the ozone is inside, I hold the animal's tail over the anus to keep the gas in. I leave the gas in for about ten minutes and then allow the animal to go out and defecate. I then take a slurry of fecal material from our super donor, mix it with saline and inject it into the same location. It's best to keep the animal from defecating for as long as possible afterward. Ozone will disrupt the biofilm, travel up the caudal rectal vein to the caudal mesenteric vein, and then travel to the liver where it stimulates the stem cells within the columnar cells in the colon. These stem cells are filled with mitochondria, and it's the action of the ozone in the mitochondria that can be a real benefit. Having the microbes mesh during sleep through a parasympathetic cycle during the night is the best.

We are using MBRT for GI problems, pancreatitis, liver and kidney inflammation, allergies, autoimmune issues, cancer, behavior, and other health concerns.

When working with the mouth microbiome, I recommend using ozonated olive oil to disrupt the biofilm and then replace it with microflora for the mouth. We call that biofilm replacement water. For over 30 years and six generations, my dogs have never had one piece of tartar, plaque, or gingivitis and have never had their teeth brushed. It is an unbalanced biofilm of the mouth that causes plaque, tartar, gingivitis, and caries.

Having ozone work to support a healthy microbiome is one of the best uses of ozone that we have in veterinary medicine.

Appendix V

Competition and Performance

This book's focus is the use of ozone therapy to treat diseases. But I want to spend a little time now discussing the use of ozone therapy to enhance performance and speed recovery after a competition. This is an exciting area because ozone is a natural substance that can be administered easily both before and after a race.

The following are ways that ozone therapy contributes to improved performance:

- Stimulates the production of antioxidants
- Increases oxygenation
- Improves body metabolism

INCREASE OF OXYGENATION

In the article "Increasing Oxygen Concentration in the Blood of the Race-horse," Dr. Barrie Sangster says, "The act of breathing is fundamental to animal life and so optimal uptake and use of oxygen is the foundation upon which equine training regimes are based. The horse's respiratory system must be fine-tuned to perform to its full potential and the skilled trainer must make himself aware of any problem which may be impeding this."

In the article, Dr. Sangster goes on to describe the respiratory process. It is helpful to understand that there are two distinct processes that can produce cellular energy. The first process is the preferred method. It is referred to as aerobic respiration. During this process, the joyful synthesis of glucose and oxygen produce adenosine triphosphate (ATP). But there is a more sinister way to produce ATP as well. In the absence of oxygen, glucose is reduced, releasing energy which drives cellular function. For short periods of time, this process can work. However, a buildup of lactic acid as a byproduct of this process can lead to muscle cramps and fatigue. Ultimately, more serious conditions can result if lack of oxygen becomes a chronic issue.

As we learned in chapter three, ozone increases the flow of oxygen across the cell membrane, which, in turn, increases oxygen levels inside of the cell. This leads to higher energy levels in the mitochondria by improving the efficiency of the respiratory chain. In red blood cells, glycolysis—the breakdown of blood sugars for cell use—is an essential process for cellular energy. An enzyme that aids in this process is phosphofructokinase. The increase of this enzyme through application of ozone to the patient also increases cellular energy (ATP) and starts a shift in the hemoglobin that enables it to offload oxygen more easily to ischemic tissues. Besides improving oxygen deliverability, ozone also improves blood flow throughout the body.

This is illustrated by a study done on the Turkish National Football League.[85] The interesting title of the study, "Doping that is not doping: Effects of ozone therapy in sportsmen," demonstrates an important point. We can safely and legally use ozone as a natural and effective way to help prepare the body for and recover from training and races. After eight weeks, the study found that the VO$_2$ max (the maximum amount of oxygen the body can utilize during exercise) increased by 16% beyond the control group, and the maximum running time was increased by 14% over the control group.

PRODUCTION OF ANTIOXIDANTS

Performance horses go through rigorous training to compete. As they train, an increase in oxygen consumption means there is a natural production of ROS in the mitochondria. It's the job of antioxidants and, in particular, glutathione, to scavenge the excess ROS, but this can prove challenging due to the sheer volume of ROS. This overproduction of ROS can cause tissue damage. We call this oxidative stress. The downstream effect of oxidative stress can be poor performance or even lameness, which is why it is critical to rid the body of ROS before they can do damage.

There have been numerous studies[86] done on the effect of supplemental antioxidants used by human athletes and competition animals to improve performance. The results have been less than impressive.[87] It seems that, instead of allowing the body to react to hormetic stressors that, in turn, produce endogenous antioxidants such as catalase, superoxide dismutase, and glutathione, the supplementation of antioxidants can keep the body from adaptation, resulting in a suppression of antioxidant production. In "Antioxidants and Exercise Performance: With a Focus on Vitamin E and C Supplementation," Higgens et al. state that "despite their negative effects on performance, free radicals may act as signaling molecules enhancing protection against greater physical stress. Current evidence suggests that antioxidant supplementation may impair these adaptations." For anyone with a working knowledge of ozone therapy, this is exactly where the lightbulb should come on. As we learned in chapter three, ozone works as a redox signaling molecule to increase antioxidant production. In the article above, we're reminded that antioxidant supplements tend to block anabolic signaling pathways, which impairs the body's ability to adapt naturally.

A 2015 study[88] published in the *Journal of Veterinary Medical Science* did a phenomenal job highlighting how ozone therapy increases antioxidant capacity. The increase peaked 3 days after the treatment and lasted for up to up to 14 days.

Summing It Up

In another study, "Daily Oxygen/O3 Treatment Reduces Muscular Fatigue and Improves Cardiac Performance in Rats Subjected to Prolonged High Intensity Physical Exercise," the authors note the hormetic effect of ozone therapy.

Hormesis is a newer area of research that studies the role of various stressors to stimulate cellular adaptation. Ultimately, the low-stress stimulus is able to precondition the cell to withstand more significant levels of stress. With ozone as the stimulant, the body responds by producing antioxidant mediators that scavenge the ROS produced during high-intensity exercise. In their study, Filippo et al. state that "they show that during a prolonged intense exercise training the rats insufflated intraperitoneally with oxygen/ozone mixture covered a higher distance per day and per week compared to the oxygen exercise trained rats. Ozone, therefore, increased the resistance of the rats to the physical fatigue and this effect was associated with modifications of physical parameters. [...] This was exerted through improvement of NO bioavailability and reduction of oxidative stress to the gastrocnemius muscle and the heart." Those physical parameters included a lower blood pressure and heart rate, lowered cardiac hypertrophy, a reduction in perivascular fibrosis in the heart, and a reduction of tissue damage biomarkers.

When you add it all together, the use of ozone therapy for competition should be a foregone conclusion.

Administration of ozone can take several forms, which have already been covered in chapter four. DIV is the easiest and fastest way to get quick results in horses, but you may not find that route acceptable. If you don't, you can administer ozone via rectal insufflation, MAHT, or intravenous ozonated saline. With smaller animals, using rectal insufflation, MAHT, or subcutaneous ozonated saline are the most common ways to administer ozone. However you choose to do it, paying attention to dosing and timing are crucial to success.

Appendix VI

Important Resources

For a complete and updated list of resources, visit
https://o3vets.com/pages/evidence.

BOOKS

- *Ozone Therapy in Veterinary Medicine* by Dr. Zullyt Zamora Rodriguez
- *Ozone. A New Medical Drug* by Velio Bocci
- *Principles and Applications of Ozone Therapy* by Dr. Frank Shallenberger
- *The Ozone Miracle* by Dr Frank Shallenberger
- *The New Oxygen Prescription* by Nathaniel Altman
- *Advances of Ozone Therapy in Medicine and Dentistry* by Dr. Sylvia Menendez

MAGAZINES AND GUIDES

- *The Madrid Declaration on Ozone Therapy*
- *The Low Dose Ozone Concept*

- *The Ozone Therapy Global Journal*
- *WFOT's Review of Evidence Based Ozone Therapy*

WEBSITES

- www.o3vets.com (Veterinary ozone therapy equipment and training)
- www.vetozonetraining.com (Ozone Therapy Training for Veterinarians)
- www.wfoot.org (World Federation of Ozone Therapy)
- www.isco3.org (International Scientific Community of Ozone Therapy)
- www.aepromo.org (Spanish Association of Medical Ozone Therapy Professionals)
- www.zotero.org/groups/46074/isco3_ozone/library (Library of articles)
- www.aaot.us (Amerian Academy of Ozone Therapy)

Meet the Author

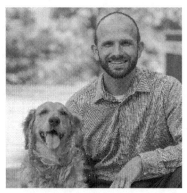

Jonathan Lowe is one of the foremost experts on ozone therapy for animals in the world and the author of the first book of its kind, *The Essential Guide to Ozone Therapy for Animals*. He is an entrepreneur, public speaker and the founder of the International Veterinary Ozone Therapy Summit – the first event of its kind designed to bring together thought leaders from around the world.

His dedication to evidence-based medicine that works in synergy with the body's biological mechanisms to bring healing is at the core of his quest to see ozone therapy become a central modality in every veterinary clinic. He is also the founder of O3Vets which received the *Innovation Award* from the Innovative Veterinary Care Journal. He resides with his wife, five children and golden retriever near Lansing, Michigan.

Notes

[1] Martin Burtscher, "Exercise limitations by the oxygen delivery and utilization systems in aging and disease: coordinated adaptation and deadaptation of the lung-heart muscle axis – a mini-review," *Gerontology*, 59, (2013):280-296.

[2] "CFR – Code of Federal Regulations Title 21," U.S. Food & Drug Administration, updated July 20, 2022: https://www.accessdata.fda.gov/scripts/cdrh/cfdocs/cfcfr/CFRSearch.cfm?fr=801.415.

[3] "Ozone Generators that are Sold as Air Cleaners," EPA, https://www.epa.gov/indoor-air-quality-iaq/ozone-generators-are-sold-air-cleaners.

[4] Yun-Gi Lee et al., "Effects of Air Pollutants on Airway Diseases," *Int J. Environ Res Public Health,* 18 (2021): 9905, https://www.ncbi.nlm.nih.gov/pmc/articles/PMC8465980/.

[5] American Meteorological Society, "Atmospheric Ozone," https://www.ametsoc.org/index.cfm/ams/about-ams/ams-statements/statements-of-the-ams-in-force/atmospheric-ozone1/.

[6] World Federation of Ozone Therapy, "WFOT's Review on Evidence Based Ozone Therapy," (2015): https://www.wfoot.org/wp-content/uploads/2016/01/WFOT-OZONE-2015-ENG.pdf.

[7] Adriana Schwartz, PhD, "Ozonotherapy History," Spanish Association Of Medical Professionals In Ozone Therapy: https://aepromo.org/en/ozonotherapy-history/.

[8] Roberto Quintero and Adriana Schwartz, "Ozone Therapy and Legislation – Analysis for Its Regularization," (2017): https://isco3.org/wp-content/uploads/2015/09/Diploma-course-Legislation-2017.pdf.

[9] A. M. Elvis and J. S. Ekta, "Ozone therapy: A clinical review," *J Nat Sci Biol Med.*, 2, (2011): 66-70, https://www.ncbi.nlm.nih.gov/pmc/articles/PMC3312702.

[10] Velio Bocci, "Is it true that ozone is always toxic? The end of a dogma," *Toxicology and Applied Pharmacology*, 3, (2006): 493-504, https://www.sciencedirect.com/science/article/pii/S0041008X06002195.

[11] M Delaville and G Thiery, "Autotransfusion with ultraviolet-irradiated blood in dogs with distemper; action of ozone on canine distemper virus and on rabbit myxomatosis virus," *Ann Pharm Fr.*, 3, (1954): 190-3, https://pubmed.ncbi.nlm.nih.gov/13171739/.

[12] Ondrej Zitka et al., "Redox status expressed as GSH:GSSG ratio as a marker for oxidative stress in paediatric tumour patients," *Oncol Lett.*, 4, (2012): 1247-1253, https://www.ncbi.nlm.nih.gov/pmc/articles/PMC3506742/.

[13] Noemi Di Marzo, Elisa Chisci, and Roberto Giovannoni, "The Role of Hydrogen Peroxide in Redox-Dependent Signaling: Homeostatic and Pathological Responses in Mammalian Cells," *Cells.*, 7, (2018): 156, https://pubmed.ncbi.nlm.nih.gov/30287799.

[14] Henry Jay Forman, Fulvio Ursini, and Matilde Maiorino, "An overview of mechanisms of redox signaling," *J Mol Cell Cardiol.*, 0, (2014): 2-9, https://www.ncbi.nlm.nih.gov/pmc/articles/PMC4048798/.

[15] O S Leon, "Ozone oxidative preconditioning: a protection against cellular damage by free radicals," *Mediators Inflamm.*, 7, (1998): 289-94, https://pubmed.ncbi.nlm.nih.gov/9792340/.

[16] Renate Viebahn-Haensler and Olga Sonia León Fernández, "Ozone in Medicine. The Low-Dose Ozone Concept and Its Basic Biochemical Mechanisms of Action in Chronic Inflammatory Diseases," *Int J Mol Sci.*, 22, (2021): 7890, https://pubmed.ncbi.nlm.nih.gov/34360655/.

[17] Noel L. Smith, "Ozone therapy: an overview of pharmacodynamics, current research, and clinical utility," *Med Gas Res.*, 7, (2017): 212-219, https://www.ncbi.nlm.nih.gov/pmc/articles/PMC5674660/.

[18] Nuo Sun, Richard J. Youle, and Toren Finkel, "The Mitochondrial Basis of Aging," *Mol Cell.*, 61, (2016): 654-666, https://www.ncbi.nlm.nih.gov/pmc/articles/PMC4779179/.

[19] V. Lobo et al., "Free radicals, antioxidants and functional foods: Impact on human health," *Pharmacogn Rev.*, 4, (2010): 118-126, https://www.ncbi.nlm.nih.gov/pmc/articles/PMC3249911/.

[20] Qiang Ma, "Role of Nrf2 in Oxidative Stress and Toxicity," *Annu Rev Pharmacol Toxicol.*, 53 (2013): 401-426, https://www.ncbi.nlm.nih.gov/pmc/articles/PMC4680839/.

[21] E B Haddad et al., "Ozone induction of cytokine-induced neutrophil chemoattractant (CINC) and nuclear factor-kappa b in rat lung: inhibition by corticosteroids ," *FEBS Lett.*, 379, (1996): 265-8, https://pubmed.ncbi.nlm.nih.gov/8603703/.

[22] Mehdi A Vostakolaei et al., "Hsp70 in cancer: A double agent in the battle between survival and death," *J Cell Physiol.*, 236, (2021): 3420-3444, https://pubmed.ncbi.nlm.nih.gov/33169384/.

[23] Catia Scassellati et al., "Ozone: a natural bioactive molecule with antioxidant property as potential new strategy in aging and in neurodegenerative disorders," *Ageing Res Rev.*, 63, (2020): 101138, https://pubmed.ncbi.nlm.nih.gov/32810649/.

[24] Toby Lawrence, "The Nuclear Factor NF-κB Pathway in Inflammation," *Cold Spring Harb Perspect Biol.*, 1, (2009): a001651, https://www.ncbi.nlm.nih.gov/pmc/articles/PMC2882124/.

[25] Anna T Grazul-Bilska et al., "Wound healing: the role of growth factors," *Drugs Today (Barc).*, 39, (2003): 787-800, https://pubmed.ncbi.nlm.nih.gov/14668934/.

[26] P. Guerra-Blanco et al., "Ozonation Degree of Vegetable Oils as the Factor of Their Anti-Inflammatory and Wound-Healing Effectiveness," *The Journal of the International Ozone Association*, 39, (2017): 374-384, https://www.tandfonline.com/doi/abs/10.1080/01919512.2017.1335185.

[27] Nathalia Rodrigues de Almeida, "Ozonized vegetable oils: Production, chemical characterization and therapeutic potential," (2016), https://www.researchgate.net/publication/318585294_Ozonized_vegetable_oils_Production_chemical_characterization_and_therapeutic_potential.

[28] Gregorio Martinez-Sanchez, "Scientific rational for the medical application of ozonized oils, an up-date," *Ozone Therapy Global Journal*, 11, (2021): 239-272, https://dialnet.unirioja.es/descarga/articulo/7943333.pdf.

[29] Adriana Simionatto Guinesi et al., "Ozonized oils: a qualitative and quantitative analysis," *Braz Dent J.*, 22, (2011): 37-40, https://pubmed.ncbi.nlm.nih.gov/21519646/.

[30] Elena Ugazio et al., "Ozonated Oils as Antimicrobial Systems in Topical Applications. Their Characterization, Current Applications, and Advances in Improved Delivery Techniques," *Molecules*, 25, (2020): 334, https://www.ncbi.nlm.nih.gov/pmc/articles/PMC7024311/.

[31] G Valacchi et al., "Ozonated oils as functional dermatological matrices: effects on the wound healing process using SKH1 mice," *Int J Pharm.*, 458, (2013): 65-73, https://pubmed.ncbi.nlm.nih.gov/24144953/.

[32] A. V. Levanov, E. E. Antipenko, and V. V. Lunin, "Primary stage of the reaction between ozone and chloride ions in aqueous solution: Can chloride ion oxidation by ozone proceed via electron transfer mechanism?," *Russian Journal of Physical Chemistry A*, 86, (2012): 584-589, https://link.springer.com/article/10.1134/S0036024412040164.

[33] Gregorio Martinez Sanchez, "Study of the ozone concentration in the ozonized saline solution," *Revista Expanola de Ozonoterapia*, 10, (2020): 55-68, https://dialnet.unirioja.es/servlet/articulo?codigo=7524335.

[34] Gregorio Martinez Sanchez, "Study of the ozone concentration in the ozonized saline solution," *Revista Expanola de Ozonoterapia*, 10, (2020): 55-68, https://dialnet.unirioja.es/servlet/articulo?codigo=7524335.

[35] Erhan Dengiz et al., "Ozone gas applied through nebulization as adjuvant treatment for lung respiratory diseases due to COVID-19 infections: a prospective randomized trial," *Med Gas Res.*, 12, (2022): 55-59, https://www.ncbi.nlm.nih.gov/pmc/articles/PMC8562398/.

[36] Zullyt Rodriguez, "*Ozone Therapy in Veterinary Medicine,*" First Edition, Collective of Authors, 2016.

[37] https://amozon.org.mx/

[38] The American Osteopathic Association of Prolotherapy Regenerative Medicine, "What is Prolotherapy?" www.prolotherapycollege.org/what-is-prolotherapy/.

[39] Wolfgang Zink and Bernhard M Graf, "Local anesthetic myotoxicity," *Reg Anesth Pain Med.*, 29, (2004): 333-40, https://pubmed.ncbi.nlm.nih.gov/15305253/.

[40] Min Seok Woo et al., "The proper concentrations of dextrose and lidocaine in regenerative injection therapy: *in vitro* study," *Korean J Pain.*, 34, (2021): 19-26, https://www.ncbi.nlm.nih.gov/pmc/articles/PMC7783851/.

[41] Geonhyeong Bae et al, "Prolotherapy for the patients with chronic musculoskeletal pain: systematic review and meta-analysis," *Anesth Pain Med (Seoul).*, 16, (2021): 81-95, https://pubmed.ncbi.nlm.nih.gov/33348947/.

[42] Frank Shallenberger, MD, HMD, ABAAM, "Prolozone™ – Regenerating Joints and Eliminating Pain," *Journal of Prolotherapy*, 3, (2011): 360-638, http://journalofprolotherapy.com/prolozone-regenerating-joints-and-eliminating-pain/.

[43] https://www.o3vets.com/wp-content/uploads/2020/11/Prolozone-Shallenberger.pdf.

[44] Masoud Hashemi et al., "The Effects of Prolotherapy With Hypertonic Dextrose Versus Prolozone (Intraarticular Ozone) in Patients With Knee Osteoarthritis," *Anesth Pain Med.*, 5, (2015): e27585, https://pubmed.ncbi.nlm.nih.gov/26587401/.

[45] Drug Crafters, "Dedicated to Improving the Health and Lives of our Patients," www.drugcrafters.com.

[46] Regina WS Sit et al., "Hypertonic dextrose injections (prolotherapy) in the treatment of symptomatic knee osteoarthritis: A systematic review and meta-analysis," *Sci Rep.*, 6, (2016): 25247, https://www.ncbi.nlm.nih.gov/pmc/articles/PMC4857084/.

[47] Ross A. Hauser et al., "A Systematic Review of Dextrose Prolotherapy for Chronic Musculoskeletal Pain," *Clin Med Insights Arthritis Musculoskelet Disord.*, 9, (2016): 139-159, https://www.ncbi.nlm.nih.gov/pmc/articles/PMC4938120/.

[48] Thrive, "Veterinary Orthopedic & Sports Medicine Group," www.vosm.com.

[49] J A McBride, "Platelet adhesiveness: the effect of centrifugation on the measurement of adhesiveness in platelet-rich plasma," *J Clin Pathol.*, 21, (1968): 397-401, https://pubmed.ncbi.nlm.nih.gov/5699080/.

[50] M J Wexler et al., "Twenty-four hour renal preservation and perfusion utilizing platelet-rich plasma," *Ann Surg.*, 174, (1971): 811-25, https://pubmed.ncbi.nlm.nih.gov/4939727/.

[51] D A Cooley et al., "Surgical treatment of aneurysms of the transverse aortic arch: experience with 25 patients using hypothermic techniques," *Ann Thorac Surg.*, 32, (1981): 260-72, https://pubmed.ncbi.nlm.nih.gov/7283518/.

[52] I. Andia et al., "Current Concepts and Translational Uses of Platelet Rich Plasma Biotechnology," *Chapter Metrics Overview*, (2014): https://www.intechopen.com/books/biotechnology/current-concepts-and-translational-uses-of-platelet-rich-plasma-biotechnology.

[53] Zheng Jun Li et al., "Autologous platelet-rich plasma: a potential therapeutic tool for promoting hair growth," *Dermatol Surg.*, 38, (2012): 1040-6, https://pubmed.ncbi.nlm.nih.gov/22455565/.

[54] Jonathan T. Ferrari and Pamela Schwartz, "Prospective Evaluation of Feline Sourced Platelet-Rich Plasma Using Centrifuge-Based Systems," *Front Vet Sci.*, 7, (2020): 322, https://www.ncbi.nlm.nih.gov/pmc/articles/PMC7303265/.

[55] Bahar Dernek and Fatma Nur Kesiktas, "Efficacy of combined ozone and platelet-rich-plasma treatment versus platelet-rich-plasma treatment alone in early stage knee osteoarthritis," *J Back Musculoskelet Rehabil.*, 32, (2019): 305-311, https://pubmed.ncbi.nlm.nih.gov/30452396/.

[56] Murat Gurger et al., "The effect of the platelet-rich plasma and ozone therapy on tendon-to-bone healing in the rabbit rotator cuff repair model," *J Orthop Surg Res.*, 16, (2021): 202, https://pubmed.ncbi.nlm.nih.gov/33740995/.

[57] Chris Cherian, Gerard Malanga, and Ken Mautner, "Optimizing Platelet-Rich Plasma (PRP) Injections: A Narrative Review," *Bio Ortho J*, 2, (2020): https://doi.org/10.22374/boj.v2i1.11.

[58] Rachita Dhurat and MS Sukesh, "Principles and Methods of Preparation of Platelet-Rich Plasma: A Review and Author's Perspective," *J*

Cutan Aesthet Surg., 7, (2014): 189-197, https://www.ncbi.nlm.nih.gov/pmc/articles/PMC4338460/.

59 Alberto Migliore and Mauro Granata, "Intra-articular use of hyaluronic acid in the treatment of osteoarthritis," *Clin INterv Aging*, 3, (2008): 365-369, https://www.ncbi.nlm.nih.gov/pmc/articles/PMC2546480/.

60 Elizaveta Kon et al., "Platelet-rich plasma intra-articular injection versus hyaluronic acid viscosupplementation as treatments for cartilage pathology: from early degeneration to osteoarthritis," *Arthroscopy*, 27, (2011): 1490-501, https://pubmed.ncbi.nlm.nih.gov/21831567.

61 Omer Mei-Dan, "Platelet-rich plasma or hyaluronate in the management of osteochondral lesions of the talus," *Am J Sports Med.*, 40, (2012): 534-41, https://pubmed.ncbi.nlm.nih.gov/22253252/.

62 John W Belk et al., "Platelet-Rich Plasma Versus Hyaluronic Acid for Knee Osteoarthritis: A Systematic Review and Meta-analysis of Randomized Controlled Trials," *Am J Sports Med.*, 49, (2021): 249-260, https://pubmed.ncbi.nlm.nih.gov/32302218/.

63 Javad Javadi Hedayatabad et al., "The Effect of Ozone (O3) versus Hyaluronic Acid on Pain and Function in Patients with Knee Osteoarthritis: A Systematic Review and Meta-Analysis," *Arch Bone Jt Surg.*, 8, (2020): 343-354, https://pubmed.ncbi.nlm.nih.gov/32766391/.

64 A Giombini et al., "Comparison between intrarticular injection of hyaluronic acid, oxygen ozone, and the combination of both in the treatment of knee osteoarthrosis," *J Biol Regul Homeost Agents.*, 30, (2016): 621-5, https://pubmed.ncbi.nlm.nih.gov/27358159/.

65 Mun-lk Lee et al., "A placebo-controlled study comparing the efficacy of intra-articular injections of hyaluronic acid and a novel hyaluronic acid-platelet-rich plasma conjugate in a canine model of

osteoarthritis," *J Orthop Surg Res.*, 14, (2019): 314, https://pub-med.ncbi.nlm.nih.gov/31533754/.

66 Evervisc, "Canine post surgical lavage," https://www.sterisanimal-health.com/media/uploads/2019/03/EV-12-EverVisc-Slick_06-15-2020.pdf.

67 https://www.vetfolio.com/learn/article/intra-articular-injections-in-dogs.

68 Jose I S Silva Junior et al., "Use of Reticulated Hyaluronic Acid Alone or Associated With Ozone Gas in the Treatment of Osteoarthritis Due to Hip Dysplasia in Dogs," *Front Vet Sci.*, 7, (2020): 265, https://pubmed.ncbi.nlm.nih.gov/32478113/.

69 Maryam Rezaie et al., "The Effect of Exercise, Ozone, and Mesenchymal Stem Cells Therapy on CB-1 and GABA Gene Expression in the Cartilage Tissue of Rats With Knee Osteoarthritis," *Pharm Biomed Res*, 6, (2020): 45-52, http://pbr.mazums.ac.ir/article-1-275-en.html.

70 Longxiang Shen et al., "The temporal effect of platelet-rich plasma on pain and physical function in the treatment of knee osteoarthritis: systematic review and meta-analysis of randomized controlled trials," *J Orthop Surg Res.*, 12, (2017): 16, https://www.ncbi.nlm.nih.gov/pmc/articles/PMC5260061/.

71 Lisa M. Billesberger, "Procedural Treatments for Knee Osteoarthritis: A Review of Current Injectable Therapies," *Pain Res Manag.*, (2020): https://www.ncbi.nlm.nih.gov/pmc/articles/PMC7049418/.

72 Yan Zhang, Feng Chen, and Song Wu, "[Clinical observation on O3 acupoint injection for treatment of low back pain]," (2007): 115-6, https://pubmed.ncbi.nlm.nih.gov/17370494/.

73 Velio Bocci, Alessandra Larini, and vanna Micheli, "Restoration of normoxia by ozone therapy may control neoplastic growth: a review and a working hypothesis," *J Altern Complement Med.*, 11, (2005): 257-65, https://pubmed.ncbi.nlm.nih.gov/15865491/.

[74] Bernardino Clavo et al., "Modulation by Ozone Therapy of Oxidative Stress in Chemotherapy-Induced Peripheral Neuropathy: The Background for a Randomized Clinical Trial," *Int J Mol Sci.*, 22, (2021): 2802, https://pubmed.ncbi.nlm.nih.gov/33802143/.

[75] T Vijayan and Jagadish G Patil, "High-tension corona controlled ozone generator for environment protection," *Journal of Physics: Conference Series*, (2010): 208, https://iopscience.iop.org/article/10.1088/1742-6596/208/1/012140/pdf.

[76] J.-S. Chang, P.A. Lawless, and T. Yamamoto, "Corona discharge processes," *IEEE Transactions on Plasma Science*, 6, (1991): 1152-1166, https://ieeexplore.ieee.org/document/125038.

[77] Absolute Ozone, "Ozone Wastewater Treatment," http://www.absoluteozone.com/ozone-generator-wastewater-treatment.html.

[78] International Ozone Association Pan American Group (PAG), "Fire Restoration," https://ioa-pag.org/Applications/Fire-Restoration.

[79] G Franke et al., "An automated room disinfection system using ozone is highly active against surrogates for SARS-CoV-2," *J Hosp Infect.*, 112, (2021): 108-113, https://pubmed.ncbi.nlm.nih.gov/33864891/.

[80] Agnieszka Joanna Brodowska, Agnieszka Nowak, and Krzysztof Smigielski, "Ozone in the food industry: Principles of ozone treatment, mechanisms of action, and applications: An overview," *Crit Rev Food Sci Nutr.*, 58, (2018): 2176-2201, https://pubmed.ncbi.nlm.nih.gov/28394634/.

[81] https://archives.federalregister.gov/issue_slice/1982/11/5/50209-50215.pdf

[82] Tara McHugh, "Ozone Processing of Foods and Beverages," (2015): https://www.ift.org/news-and-publications/food-technology-magazine/issues/2015/november/columns/processing.

[83] Larissa Vivan Cestonaro et al., "Ozone generated by air purifier in low concentrations: friend or foe?" *Environ Sci Pollut Res Int.*, 24, (2017): 22673-22678, https://pubmed.ncbi.nlm.nih.gov/28812184/.

[84] *Lancet*, 399, (2022): 629-655, https://pubmed.ncbi.nlm.nih.gov/35065702/.

[85] Mustafa Tansel Turan, "Doping that it not a doping. Effects of ozone therapy in sportmen." *Journal of Ozone Therapy*, 5, (2021): https://ojs.uv.es/index.php/JO3T/article/view/21386.

[86] Rebecca J Marshall et al., "Supplemental vitamin C appears to slow racing greyhounds," *J Nutr.*, 132, (2002): 1616S-21S, https://pubmed.ncbi.nlm.nih.gov/12042473/.

[87] Madalyn Riley Higgins, Azimeh Izadi, and Mojtaba Kaviani, "Antioxidants and Exercise Performance: With a Focus on Vitamin E and C Supplementation," *Int J Environ Res Public Health*, 17, (2020): 8452, https://pubmed.ncbi.nlm.nih.gov/33203106/.

[88] Nao TSUZUKI et al., "Effects of ozonated autohemotherapy on the antioxidant capacity of Thoroughbred horses," *J Vet Med Sci.*, 77, (2015): 1647-1650, https://www.ncbi.nlm.nih.gov/pmc/articles/PMC4710722/.

Made in United States
Troutdale, OR
10/26/2023

14024128R10116